The Vital Questions Series

CLEAR THINKING FOR FAITHFUL LIVING

□ □

These books investigate key issues that make a practical difference in how Christians think and act. The goal is to provide a substantial, accessible discussion of issues about which Christians need to know more. This series is intended as a service to the church and to individuals with the aim of better preparing a "Christian mind," resulting in more faithful living.

Daniel Taylor, General Editor

□ □

This book is a project of The Center for Bioethics and Human Dignity, an international center located just north of Chicago, Illinois, in the United States of America. The Center brings Christian perspectives to bear on today's many pressing bioethical challenges such as those addressed in this book. It pursues this task by developing three book series, nine audio series, nine video series, numerous conferences in different parts of the world, and a variety of other printed and computer-based resources.

Each July the Center offers a cutting-edge national/international conference and week-long bioethics training institutes for which continuing education and graduate or undergraduate academic credit are available. In fact, it is possible today for people to earn a master's degree in bioethics, in one or more years, without relocating from their current home or job.

Through its membership/support program, the Center networks and provides resources for people interested in bioethical matters all over the world. Members/supporters receive the Center's international journal, *Ethics and Medicine,* the Center's newsletter, *Dignity,* special Center communications, an Internet news service, and discounts on all Center resources and events.

For more information on membership in the Center or its various resources, contact:

THE CENTER FOR **BIOETHICS** AND HUMAN DIGNITY

The Center for Bioethics and Human Dignity
2065 Half Day Road
Bannockburn, IL 60015 USA
Phone: (847) 317-8180
Fax: (847) 317-8101
E-mail: info@cbhd.org

Topical information, today's news, and ordering are available through the Center's Internet Web site: www.cbhd.org.

□ □

Does God Need Our Help?

Cloning, Assisted Suicide,
& Other Challenges in Bioethics

□ □ □ □ □ □ *JOHN F. KILNER and C. BEN MITCHELL*
DANIEL TAYLOR, GENERAL EDITOR

Tyndale House Publishers, Inc., Wheaton, Illinois

Visit Tyndale's exciting Web site at www.tyndale.com

Does God Need Our Help? Cloning, Assisted Suicide, and Other Challenges in Bioethics

Copyright © 2003 by John F. Kilner and C. Ben Mitchell. All rights reserved.

Cover art copyright © 2002 by Getty Images. All rights reserved.

Designed by Kelly Bennema and Luke Daab

Edited by Daniel Taylor and MaryLynn Layman

Unless otherwise indicated, all Scripture quotations are taken from the *Holy Bible,* New International Version®. NIV®. Copyright © 1973, 1978, 1984 by International Bible Society. Used by permission of Zondervan Publishing House. All rights reserved.

Scripture quotations marked KJV are taken from the *Holy Bible,* King James Version.

Scripture quotations marked NLT are taken from the *Holy Bible,* New Living Translation, copyright © 1996. Used by permission of Tyndale House Publishers, Inc., Wheaton, Illinois 60189. All rights reserved.

Scripture quotation marked NRSV are taken from the New Revised Standard Version of the Bible, copyright © 1989 by the Division of Christian Education of the National Council of the Churches of Christ in the United States of America, and are used by permission. All rights reserved.

Library of Congress Cataloging-in-Publication Data

Kilner, John Frederic.

 Does God need our help? : cloning, assisted suicide, and other challenges in bioethics / John F. Kilner and C. Ben Mitchell.
  p. cm. — (Vital questions)
Includes bibliographical references and index.
 ISBN 0-8423-7446-9
 1. Medical ethics—Religious aspects—Christianity. 2. Bioethics—Religious aspects—Christianity. 3. Christian ethics. I. Mitchell, C. Ben. II. Title. III. Vital questions (Tyndale House Publishers)
R725.56 .K548 2003
179.7—dc21   2003001366

Printed in the United States of America

07   06   05   04   03
 7   6   5   4   3   2   1

Contents

10. Remaking Humans: The New Utopians versus a
    Truly Human Future 191

Acknowledgments

This is not another academic book. Much too often members of academic disciplines write for the benefit of their academic peers. Whether in law, medicine, philosophy, science, or theology, we tend to write for one another.

The challenge of leaving the comfortable confines of the vocabulary and categories of one's discipline can be daunting. Yet, the issues of bioethics demand our best effort. Why? Because bioethics is about us all. We all make decisions about birth, death, and the life in between. The writer of Ecclesiastes expresses this truth for us all when he says: "For everything there is a season, and a time for every matter under heaven: a time to be born and a time to die" (Ecclesiastes 3:1-2, NRSV).

It is our hope that this book will be useful to those who must make decisions about life and death. Every page was written with the view that people will use this as a tool to help them or their family members make some of the most important decisions they will ever make. That is sobering.

We also recognize that some of the most signifi-

cant decisions about the ways technology devel-
ops will be made by society at large. How crucial
it is for a Christian perspective to inform those decisions! That will not happen, though, unless a
whole range of people understand what insights a
Christian perspective contributes. We offer this
book as one way to promote such understanding.

While we take responsibility for any of the
shortcomings of the book, we must express our
deepest thanks to those who helped us by re-
viewing the manuscript. E. David Cook, of Oxford University, and Arthur Holmes Professor of
Faith and Learning at Wheaton College, gave us
very helpful suggestions. We also wish to thank
his colleague David Fletcher, associate professor
of philosophy at Wheaton. Needless to say, the
non-academics who provided helpful critique
were especially important in the development of
this book. Special thanks in this regard to Erwin
Jacobsen and MaryLynn Layman.

Series editor Dan Taylor offered extraordinary
assistance and has been a joy to work with. Both
our wives, who are invested in our work as much
as we are, helped us remember our audience.
Thank you, Suzanne and Nancy.

Ultimately, the proof of the pudding is in the eating. So we hope you, the reader, find this volume useful as you face difficult bedside decisions and biotech challenges. At the end of the book you will find a list of resources to assist you in delving deeper into each area.

Introduction
Why All the Fuss?

The world we pass on to our children and their children may be dazzlingly wonderful or staggeringly horrible.

Michelle, for one, will be healed. She is a teenager who endures a life of stomach pain, vomiting, aching joints, skin sores, and the progressive breakdown of her blood. She has sickle-cell anemia, a disabling and potentially fatal disease. Its cause is a small mistake in her genetic code, which will eventually be correctable. In fact, because of genetic and other technologies, many of the worst diseases you have heard about and may be experiencing in your own family will be cured!

At the same time, David and Maria may wake up one morning horrified at what they have done. It started out fairly innocently, or so they thought. They had aborted their second child because they didn't want another boy. Then they had tried a new genetic intervention technique to ensure that the next child would be a girl, and at the same time they took advantage of the chance to boost the girl's mental and physical abilities. But a genetic error had caused the baby's right arm not to develop properly, and they decided to abort her as well. Two additional pregnancies resulted in similar deformities and more abortions. Since then Maria hasn't been able to get pregnant again. Now the morning newspaper is saying that the use of genetic "improvement" techniques were approved too quickly—resulting in deformities in children and infertility in women.

In other words, with the wonder comes a warning. It is expressed well by Bill Joy, the chief scientist of one of Silicon Valley's top technology companies and cochairman of a U.S. presidential commission on the future of information technology: "We are being propelled into this new century with no plan, no control, no brakes." Even worse, he adds, "The last chance to assert control—the failsafe point—is rapidly approaching."[1] If this warning were from some paranoid fanatic with no real knowledge of the issues, it would be one thing. But Bill Joy is a respected leader in cutting-edge technology.

What will make the difference in which way the future goes? Bioethics will. *Bioethics?* What's that? Simply put, bioethics involves distinguishing between what we should pursue and shouldn't pursue in matters of life and health. For example, we know having babies is a good thing, but would it be a good option to produce them through cloning? Would it be okay not just to make them a copy of another person, but to engineer them to be exactly the way we want them to be? The human race—that's you, plus everyone you know, plus others—must decide very soon what to pursue and what not to pursue. We need to decide long before the economic interests get too heavily involved and changing direction is virtually impossible.

If we truly can make such a difference in the future, then why in the world have we not all become *bioethicists*? Or why are we not all at least engaging these issues in our private and public lives in whatever ways we can?

Two reasons stand out. First, we are simply not aware of how huge and radically important the issues racing toward us are. This book is designed to help remedy that information gap. In part 3 of this volume, you will find chapters not only on reproductive, cloning, and genetic technologies, which are interventions you probably have heard something about but may not really understand; you will also find information on such developments as *cybernetics* and *nanotechnology,* which you may have thought were pure science fiction—if you've heard about them at all.

What do you think about a computer chip implanted in your brain to give you a vast storehouse of information and even a live connection to the Internet (viruses included)? How about self-reproducing machines too small to see that can attack germs (or healthy tissue) in our bodies? Both are doable—but does "can do" mean "should do"?

There is a second important reason that we fail to make bioethics a priority. We simply don't realize that the decisions we already make concerning our health and lives are basically *bioethical* ones. If our dying mother or father needs one last medical treatment, we consider the decision to be purely medical and so ask our doctor to tell us what should be done. Or if we want to pursue one of thirty-eight options for having children when we are infertile, we consider choosing the right option to be a decision for a fertility specialist to make.

Wrong. We do need the best medical counsel we can get in such situations. But identifying the best decision will also require recognizing what is at stake *ethically* in each option before us. You may be told, for instance, that the use of dialysis to filter the impurities from your dying spouse's blood would not be worthwhile. Rather, it would simply be best to provide good pain relief and emotional support. But what does "worthwhile" mean? Your spouse may have a quality of life on dialysis that a physician or administrator does not consider to be worth the cost of treatment. You or your spouse may think otherwise were you to have all of the information.

How much should you be told? What role should you play in the treatment decision? How different might you and a particular physician be in the value you each place on human life? People should be getting the best medical information available concerning all possible options and then tracking down the best possible ethical information for the situation. Both are necessary to be fully equipped to make good decisions. But people rarely leave the confines of the hospital. (Of course, those blessed with a Christian physician may not have to, *if* the physician can provide patients with the bioethical as well as medical information they need.)

On the other hand, a close friend or family member may be diagnosed with infertility. Perhaps she receives medical counsel to pursue *in vitro* fertilization (fertilizing her eggs in the lab and then implanting the resulting embryos in her womb). The process may be described to her for her to approve, and she may be pleased that she has been informed and even consulted for her approval. No ethical dilemmas here, right?

Look again. Did you know that it is not medically necessary to have many eggs fertilized in order to end up with an embryo to implant? Did you know that the number is so high in order to improve the odds of a successful pregnancy that some embryonic human beings—your loved one's newly conceived children—will almost certainly die as a result? What significance does an early embryo have, and how does a risk to an embryo compare with a risk of not giving birth at all? People should be getting the best medical information they can and then hunting down their clergy or other well-informed Christian leaders to get the ethical information they need just as much. But they rarely do, either because they see the issue as purely medical rather than ethical, or because they see Christian leaders as unlikely to have useful bioethical resources available.

This must change. If we do not recognize today's bioethical issues of life and death clamoring for attention all around us, we will likely remain unaware of tomorrow's as well. Today many individuals, including our loved ones, will suffer as a result. Tomorrow the entire human race will be in jeopardy.

But what a different picture is possible if we recognize the issues and know how to engage them! People can live and die well, with the confidence that God is pleased with the choices they are making. Health care professionals can be a welcome source of information and counsel in the decision-making process. Elderly, embryonic, and other persons, instead of being "used" for the benefit of others, can be respected as the human beings they are—created in the image of God.

Part 2 of this book is designed to help foster such a world. Chapter 4 focuses on matters with special significance for human embryos, such as stem cell research and abortion. The next chapter addresses end-of-life challenges, such as withholding and withdrawing treatment, and how such decisions differ from resource allocation decisions with which they are often confused. Part 2 closes with a discussion of the temptations of assisted suicide and euthanasia.

Part 3 then goes beyond more familiar health care issues to grapple with some major, emerging biotech issues: reproductive, cloning, and genetic technologies. It ends with a chapter discussing the growing battle over whether or not we should be employing biotechnology to remake the human race into a "new improved version"— or even to replace humans entirely.

Before diving into the specific issues of health care and biotechnology, however, this book takes seriously the need for bioethical tools. We cannot possibly address here every situation that you will encounter. But we can provide you with some tools that will serve you well in any situation.

Three tools are especially useful, and each receives a chapter in Part 1: history, ethics, and the Bible. History tells us where we come from and who, as a result, we are. Health care today is desperately in need of clarity on these points. Ethics alerts us to how much more is involved than medical information in deciding how we ought to live. The Bible gives us a compass to provide direction in the face of many options. To supplement these tools, the book concludes with a discussion of other important bioethical resources available today.

We cannot wait much longer to become informed and engaged. People all around us are experiencing great bioethical challenges from the beginning to the end of their lives. Meanwhile, the lure of commercial profits is attracting vast resources to underwrite biotech research. We must not underestimate the danger if we do not formulate ethical guidelines for the development and use of emerging biotechnologies.

Imagine the grief of the parents of the patient at a major U.S. university medical center who was not expected to die soon, but who abruptly died in a genetic therapy experiment. Their lawsuit suggests they are convinced that they were given inadequate warnings because of the pressures to push ahead with the research as quickly as possible. If we wait too long to develop better safeguards, it will be like waiting until after a flood has occurred to try to dig a channel to direct the floodwaters in a productive direction. The time to design and dig the channel is before the flood hits!

Think of those who were living in the years leading up to the *Roe v. Wade* U.S. Supreme Court decision that opened the door to legal abortion. Very few took notice of what surely was coming until after it came. May that not be said of our generation in the face of a much larger array of vital bioethical challenges.

PART ONE

□ □ □ □ □

TOOLS:
Distinguishing
Right from Wrong

It Started with Hippocrates

With purity and with holiness I will pass my life and practice my Art.

HIPPOCRATES

Almost everyone has heard of the Hippocratic Oath, the ancient pledge sworn by newly minted physicians. Few people know just what the Oath says and even fewer know that many medical schools no longer require their graduates to take the Oath. Since the ethics expounded in the Oath have shaped the course of Western medicine for over 2,500 years, it is important for us to understand something of the history and contents of the Oath. We must also understand the challenges physicians face—especially Christian physicians—as they try to maintain fidelity to the principles and virtues outlined in what may be called the "Hippocratic consensus" in medicine. Biomedical ethics did not rise phoenixlike from the ashes of the twentieth century. In fact, like medicine, biomedical ethics has ancient beginnings.

Some form of medicine has existed since at least 9000 B.C. The historical evidence suggests that the first physicians were really priestly magicians whose treatments and cures arose from their cultic practices rather than scientific research. The practice of medicine consisted largely of spells, incantations, charms, and a few natural drugs given to patients as part of a spell to rid them of an ailment. Many of these treatments may have been helpful, though one must wonder whether some of the patients might have been better off without treatment.

In Mesopotamia three classes of physicians existed: the diviners (who interpreted omens and foretold the course of diseases), the exorcists (who cast out the evil spirits believed to have caused the disease), and the physicians (who performed surgery and administered drugs). The Code of Hammurabi (ca. 2000 B.C.), an ancient law code, spelled out some of the protocols to be followed in Babylonian medicine. For example, if a physician treated a nobleman for a severe wound or for an abscessed eye and the nobleman either died or lost his eye, the physician's hands should be cut off! These laws, no doubt, made the idea of becoming a doctor less attractive to prospective physicians. The Code included little, if anything, that could be described as ethics.

Early Western Medicine

Western scientific medicine really began with the Greeks. Though some Egyptian medical practices were transferred to Greece, Hellenistic culture can be credited with much of our early knowledge of anatomy, physiology, and the genesis of our medical terminology. Even the symbol of medicine, the caduceus—the familiar serpent entwined on a rod—probably owes its origin to the Greek deities Aesculapius and Hermes, as well as the cult of the serpent in Minoan religion. Other Greek giants such as Aristotle, Galen, and Hippocrates shaped medicine in innumerable ways.

Hippocrates of Cos (ca. 460–ca. 370 B.C.) was the son of a physician and practiced as an itinerant doctor in Thrace, Thessaly, and Macedonia. Plato mentions Hippocrates in the *Phaedrus,* where Socrates appeals to the empirical observations of Hippocrates and the Asclepiad, the cult of Aesculapius. Plato also calls Hippocrates "a professional trainer of medical students."[1]

The written works attributed to Hippocrates

are of various origins. Some are doubtless the works of Hippocrates himself. *Prognostics* and *Joints* are usually thought to be original. Other works were written under his name either by individuals or by the so-called Hippocratic school. The Hippocratic corpus of some sixty written works is rich and varied. His *Aphorisms,* for instance, begins: "Life is short, and the Art long; the occasion fleeting; experience fallacious, and judgment difficult. The physician must not only be prepared to do what is right himself, but also to make the patient, the attendants, and externals co-operate."[2]

The Hippocratic Oath

Hippocrates is perhaps best known to most of us through the Oath that bears his name. What has become known as the Hippocratic Oath was probably written after his death by the Hippocratic school. Nevertheless, the Oath is universally held to reflect accurately the ethics of Hippocrates himself.

Originally the Oath was not recited in medical schools. Rather, it was administered in family guilds of physicians or used to form a pact between a teacher and his pupil.

Jews, Christians, and Muslims adopted the Oath as their own, changing the names of the Greek deities to the names of Yahweh and Allah, respectively, thus making the Oath monotheistic rather than polytheistic.

The purpose of the Oath

When thinking about the purpose of the Oath, it is important to remember that in Hippocrates' day there were no medical schools, examination boards, or professional organizations that offered credentials to physicians. No training was required, no licensure was necessary, and no one could, therefore, remove a physician from practice. Medicine was considered a craft and the physician was a craftsman.

Anyone could (and did) hang out a shingle, as it were, and call himself a physician. (In the ancient world physicians were, almost without exception, males.) As we have noted, not only were some of the physicians the equivalent of sorcerers, but there were plenty of charlatans who took advantage of the sick for their own profit. The patient had to be able to distinguish the charlatan from the true physician.

The Hippocratic school was probably like a

crafts guild. A Hippocratic physician demonstrated mastery over a particular set of skills. Many of the works that bear the name of Hippocrates outlined those skills. The Hippocratic physician was also held to high ethical standards. These standards are expounded clearly in the Oath itself.

> I swear by Apollo the physician and Aesculapius, and Health, and All-heal, and all the gods and goddesses, that, according to my ability and judgment,
>
> I will keep this Oath and this stipulation—to reckon him who taught me this Art equally dear to me as my parents, to share my substance with him, and relieve his necessities if required; to look upon his offspring in the same footing as my own brothers, and to teach them this art, if they shall wish to learn it, without fee or stipulation; and that by precept, lecture, and every other mode of instruction,
>
> I will impart a knowledge of the Art to my own sons, and those of my teachers, and to disciples bound by a stipulation and oath according to the law of medicine, but to none others.

I will follow that system of regimen which, according to my ability and judgment, I consider for the benefit of my patients, and abstain from whatever is deleterious and mischievous.

I will give no deadly medicine to anyone if asked, nor suggest any such counsel; and in like manner I will not give to a woman a pessary to produce abortion. With purity and with holiness I will pass my life and practice my Art.

I will not cut persons labouring under the stone, but will leave this to be done by men who are practitioners of this work. Into whatever houses I enter, I will go into them for the benefit of the sick, and will abstain from every voluntary act of mischief and corruption; and, further, from the seduction of females or males, of freemen and slaves. Whatever, in connection with my professional service, or not in connection with it, I see or hear, in the life of men, which ought not to be spoken of abroad,

I will not divulge, as reckoning that all such should be kept secret. While I continue to keep this Oath unviolated, may it be granted to me to enjoy life and the practice of the Art, respected

by all men, in all times. But should I trespass and
violate this Oath, may the reverse be my lot.

The Oath divides neatly into two parts: the
first specifies the duties of the pupil toward his
teacher, and the second provides a brief summary
of the ethics of medicine. In the first part it is evident that being a physician was much like being
any other kind of craftsman.

Certain duties were required of the learner of a
craft toward his teacher. First, upon entering
training for medicine, the student was to treat the
master as he would his own father, even supporting the teacher should that become necessary.
This was a form of indenture, but a more intimate
form than others in the ancient world. For in this
indenture, the offspring of the teacher were to be
regarded as siblings of the student. Moreover, the
student pledged to teach the master's children
the art of medicine should they wish to learn it.

Surprisingly, the student also covenanted to
teach other pupils who signed the indenture and
swore the Physicians' Law (another term for the
Oath), "but to none other." As Nigel Cameron has
pointed out in his very helpful volume, *The New
Medicine: Life and Death After Hippocrates,* "The

Oath explicitly forbids the physician to pass on his clinical knowledge to anyone who has not already committed himself to the Hippocratic values."[3] The skills of clinical medicine were only to be taught to those who would embrace the ethics of medicine.

The Ethics of the Oath

What are Hippocratic ethics? In another place in the Hippocratic literature Hippocrates says, "The medical art has to consider three factors, the disease, the patient, and the physician. The physician is the servant of his art, and the patient must cooperate with the doctor in combating the disease."[4] These three factors—the disease, the patient, and the physician—clearly inform the moral requirements of being a physician.

First, the Oath is written against the backdrop of the patient's disease. The patient is sick. The patient has a disease that requires the physician's skills to treat. Following the outline of the Oath, the disease may require a change of diet, the administration of drugs, or surgery. In the application of all these treatments, the primary concern is for the good of the patient. He or she is the focus of the Hippocratic physician's art. The physician serves his art to the end that the patient's sickness is relieved.

Also, note carefully that the Oath enjoins the physician to employ his skills "for the benefit" of the patient and in such a way as not to be "deleterious and mischievous." It is a well-known axiom that the first principle of medical ethics is *primum non nocere* (first, do no harm). After that, the physician is also to seek to do good for his patient by skillfully and competently treating the patient's illness.

It is a well-known axiom that the first principle of medical ethics is *primum non nocere* (first, do no harm).

Doing no harm means, among other things, that the physician will not give a poison to anyone or even make a suggestion to that effect. Physician-assisted suicide is beyond the pale of "purity and holiness" for the Hippocratic physician.

Similarly, doing no harm means that the physician will not give an abortion-causing drug to one of his female patients. Abortion was not uncommon in the Graeco-Roman world. Nevertheless, the Hippocratic physician was to set himself apart from this practice, no matter how common it might be. Interestingly, in one Christianized version of the Oath the language is even more explicit, stating that the physician will refuse to perform an abortion "from above or below." This would prohibit both the use of drugs or surgery for the purposes of abortion—once again underscoring the fact that early Christians knew abortion to be a common cultural practice.

Further, the Hippocratic physician pledges not to practice beyond his competence. Thus, he swore that he would refer patients with a "stone" to a surgeon. Here we have an ancient testimony to the emergence of specialties in medicine. Apparently there were already what we call internists and surgeons.

Next, we should observe that the Hippocratic physician was a "professional." That is to say, there was no dichotomy between his "life" and his "art." A professional is ideally a thoroughly integrated individual who is on the inside just what one sees on the outside.

Professionalism means that he will keep himself from wrongdoing, including sexual immorality

> **We** should observe that the Hippocratic physician was a "professional"; there was no dichotomy between his "life" and his "art."

of either a heterosexual or homosexual nature. Sexual sin is especially heinous where a person of considerable power (in this case the physician with his special set of skills and expertise) is in a position to exploit a person who is weaker (in this case due both to the presence of an illness and by the social structures of the day).

Moreover, the professionalism of the physician means that he will keep confidential any information about the patient and/or information learned during the treatment of the patient. Patient confidentiality is no less important today for some of the same reasons it was important in Hippocrates' era. Patients can easily be discriminated against based on their diagnoses and prognoses. If someone does learn of a patient's condition, it should not be, says the Oath, from the physician.

Finally, the Oath ends with a sanction showing its utter seriousness. The consequences of keeping the Oath were to be a life of flourishing and respect. If the physician violated his covenant, he called down misery and disapproval on himself.

Evidence of the sober nature of the Oath was that it was pledged in the name of the gods. While Christians obviously will not name the pagan deities when they pledge the Oath, they nonetheless recognize, as Hippocrates recognized, that the practice of medicine is transcendent in nature.

Human beings are not merely creatures of flesh and blood; they are spiritual and "soulish" creatures. Moreover, the universe is more than a merely physical universe. So the task of caring for patients compromised by illness must be performed in light of realities that go beyond the physical.

The Costs of Ignoring the Oath

The Hippocratic Oath enshrined the ideals of medical practice in the Western world. Much of what we think of as medicine and medical ethics is derived from the Hippocratic tradition. Christians modified the Oath in important ways. They did not, however, dilute the Oath. They only strengthened it. Today, medicine is changing. We are jettisoning many of the Hippocratic, not to mention Christian, ideals. We do so at our own peril and, more importantly, at the peril of those who are sick.

> **The Hippocratic Oath enshrined the ideals of medical practice in the Western world.**

In a very important survey of medical schools in North America in the mid-1990s, Robert Orr,

M.D., and his colleagues found that only one medical school of the 157 surveyed used the original Hippocratic Oath. Sixty-eight schools used some version of the Oath, but only 8 percent of those oaths prohibited abortion and only 14 percent prohibited assisted suicide and euthanasia.[5]

Orr and his colleagues also found that while 100 percent of the oaths taken in North American medical schools included an affirmation of the physician's commitment to the patient's well-being, only 43 percent included the notion of accountability for the physician's own actions and only 3 percent prohibited sexual contact with patients.[6] These distortions of the Oath reflect gargantuan changes in the ethics of medicine.

There is a stark contrast between Hippocratic medicine and contemporary, relativistic medicine. In a very real sense, the remainder of this book is a plea for a revival of the principles and values resident in the Judeo-Christian Hippocratic tradition in medicine. Human life and dignity are on the line.

2 Then Along Came Bioethics

As we began to see in the previous chapter, the ethical outlook of Hippocrates that launched and guides the medical profession is substantially ignored by many today. Yet there is so much attention devoted to ethics in medicine today. How can these both be true?

The answer is rooted in the two different roles that ethics can play. One role helps us understand the way things are, and the other helps us understand the way things ought to be. In either case, ethics is about distinguishing between good and bad, between right and wrong. So the first role for ethics is to help us understand the various ways people *actually* determine who they should be and what they should do. The second role of ethics is to tell us the *best* way to do this.

When "bio" is added to the front of the word *ethics,* it signals that issues of life and health are in view. Although *bioethics* could therefore refer to environmental issues in addition to matters of health care and biotechnology, it more commonly focuses on the latter two arenas. Those two are also the focus of this book.

Hippocratic ethics is a good example of the second role that bioethics can play. It tells us how everyone ought to behave in matters of life and health. Because the biblically informed Judeo-Christian worldview recognizes a similar set of ethical norms applicable to everyone, it has been quite compatible with Hippocratic ethics. Furthermore, because so many people in Western civilization have affirmed these outlooks, they have served as almost unconscious guides to ethical living, particularly in medicine. In recent centuries, even the prevailing non-Christian secular outlook has affirmed that there is a set of ethical norms applicable to everyone.

During the last decades of the twentieth century, however, with the rise of so-called "postmodernism," that basic notion of ethics applicable to all was radically questioned in every sphere of life, including health care. As a result, fewer and fewer people had an intuitive set of convictions that directed our life together. Various fields of "ethics" such as bioethics and business ethics arose to help us identify our options. This is the first role of bioethics noted above. It helps us identify and evaluate the various ways that people think we ought to provide health care and use biotechnology. This is indeed an important task if we are to engage today's world, and it is the focus of this chapter.

However, bioethics can do more than merely discuss options. Secular bioethics may be increasingly unable to do more than this, at least to the extent that it rests on the assumption there is no such thing as "truth" or "absolute right and wrong" that applies to everyone.

Bioethics helps us identify and evaluate the various ways that people think we ought to provide health care and use biotechnology.

However, bioethics from a Christian perspective not only can critically evaluate the ways that people justify their actions, but also can explain how people ought to live. For all people have been created by God, in God's own image, to have certain aspects of life in common. To be sure, people and their circumstances are different in many ways, and how they ought to live will vary in many respects. But, biblically, there are certain core ethical guides that all must live by if they are to flourish. What this unity within diversity means for bioethics will be the subject of chapter 3.

More Than Reasoning

The first role of bioethics, then, is to help us understand the various ways people determine who they should be and what they should do. It is easy to assume that people take different ethical positions on issues of life and health because they justify their positions differently. One person does what will produce the best consequences; another does what the rules require, and so forth. However, there is much more to it than that.

Researchers have studied thousands of bioethical disagreements over issues such as abortion. It turns out that, when people come to different ethical conclusions, it is for one of four reasons: There is a difference in facts, beliefs, loyalties, or reasoning. Two people may be similar in three of these four areas, but a significant difference in one of them alone can result in the two people taking different positions on a bioethical issue.

Consider a difference in *facts*. Facts are what can be identified and measured by our physical senses. For example, they can be seen, heard, smelled, tasted, and/or felt. In the abortion debate, they include the genetic and biological makeup of a fetus, as well as the risk to the mother's health and life posed by each abortion procedure. It is not hard to see how people could come to different conclusions if they are working with different facts. A person may be convinced that some women will die unless they can use a particular abortion procedure. Such a person will be much more likely to support the use of that procedure in those cases than a person who is convinced that the women are not at risk.

A difference in *beliefs* functions in much the same way. Beliefs are convictions people have that go beyond what our physical senses can verify. It is important to note here that they are not necessarily any less true than facts. They simply are acquired differently. They include what we know by faith rather than by sight alone (to use the biblical categories of 2 Corinthians 5:7). But beliefs are not necessarily religious in nature. They include people's intuitions about the way the world is or ought to be. They even include people's *interpretation* of what the facts in a particular situation *mean*. In the abortion debate, beliefs include convictions about the significance of the fetus. Two people may agree about the biological description of the fetus. But one may see that fetus as ultimately the result of a random combination of molecules followed by a natural evolutionary process. The other may see that same fetus as a creation of God, reflecting the very image of God. As a result, the second person may be much less likely to abort a fetus than the first.

The relevance of *loyalties* here may be less evident, but their influence on our bioethical views is no less significant. Loyalties are attachments we have, to someone or something, that cause us to think or behave in certain ways. We may have loyalties to family, to a political party, to a religious group, and so forth. Where such a loyalty exists, we may steadfastly take a particular position on abortion, for instance, simply because those to whom we are loyal take that position.

There is one form of loyalty, though, that is far more subtle and yet more widespread than any other. It is our loyalty to ourselves. Because of our sinful, self-centered natures (see chapter 3), we tend to give extra weight to how things will affect us personally. Accordingly, two people may be operating with the same facts, beliefs, and forms of reasoning, but they may come to different conclusions about how ethical a particular abortion is because of a personal stake one has in the outcome.

The form of *reasoning* we use determines how we take all of the facts, beliefs, and loyalties and reach a conclusion from them. Different ways we can do this are discussed below. However, what we need to see first is that our bioethical views are not simply the result of our reasoning—that is, how we think. It is important to take a look at the way we think because that is often the source of our differences on bioethical issues. But we must also be on the lookout for differences in the factual understanding, beliefs, and loyalties that people bring to a particular situation.

When we seek to persuade others of our position, and there are significant differences in factual understanding, we must attempt to reach an agreement with them about what the facts really are. If they recognize they have misunderstood the facts, they may well change their position— just as we should be open to changing ours if it turns out that we have misunderstood the facts!

Where there are relevant differences in beliefs and loyalties, several approaches are possible. We can attempt to persuade others to adopt our beliefs and loyalties. Alternately, we can try to explain why a particular belief or loyalty need not commit someone to a particular position on the bioethical issue at hand.

For example, suppose that someone's religious community holds that trust in God means refusing lifesaving antibiotics in a particular situation. It may be possible to show how a person can be faithful to that religious community's reverence for God without refusing the antibiotics. Again, such discussions can sometimes help *us* recognize where we have beliefs or loyalties that are not biblically sound and should be adjusted!

Reasoning Matters

Often, though, when people disagree over a bioethical issue, it is because they take different approaches to reasoning, perhaps unconsciously. As indicated above, reasoning simply refers to the way we take all of the relevant information, such as facts, beliefs, and loyalties, and reach a conclusion from them. There are many ways that people do this, but three methods are most common. Some people appeal to consequences, others to principles, and still others to virtues.

One of the most influential ways to justify our

views and actions involves appealing to their *consequences*. Whatever action or behavior will bring the most benefit to the most people is the right thing to do. John Stuart Mill captured the key idea here in his famous slogan "the greatest good for the greatest number." What could be more ethically praiseworthy than benefiting people? If the benefit is as great as possible, and reaches as many people as possible, so much the better. Current examples abound, as we will see in later chapters. For instance, embryonic stem cell research promises to produce cures for many medical problems, so some would say that it must therefore be good.

> **R**easoning simply refers to the way we take all of the relevant information, such as facts, beliefs, and loyalties, and reach a conclusion from them.

As attractive as this way of thinking appears, it is unworkable in practice, if we are honest; and it is dangerous as well. It is unworkable for more than one reason. First, if the right decision depends on how everyone is affected, then we must be able to identify how any action we take will ultimately affect all people in the world who can be affected by it, now and far into the future. In fact, the impact on all future generations must also be taken into account. When we recognize the impossibility of such a task, we can appreciate the man who moaned, "God may be a consequentialist, but people can't be—they don't have the infinite knowledge necessary!"

A bioethics of consequences is also unworkable because it requires us to use the same unit—dollars, pleasurable feelings, or something else—to measure every consequence so that we can compare them all. But there is no such unit. Is the benefit you would receive at the end of your life from living one day longer worth $127? $128? 19.46 "units" of pleasure? How would that benefit compare with the benefit your neighbors receive from the piece of art displayed in the local city hall?

The impossibility of knowing and measuring every consequence precisely means that consequence-oriented people simply take into account whatever information they have easiest access to and give it whatever weight strikes them as appropriate. Right and wrong then become merely a product of each person's location and biases, differing from one person to the next. We are left with no real right and wrong, just personal preferences.

This open door to bias begins to suggest why attempting to justify our actions purely by their consequences is not only unworkable but also dangerous. It subjects some individuals and minority groups to serious harm. If someone wants to achieve benefits by abusing or oppressing certain people, there is nothing wrong, according to this approach, with doing so. There are no limits in this way of thinking to what can be done to an individual or group in order to produce good consequences. The negative impact on some will have to be taken into account. But if enough people benefit sufficiently as a result, then the ends justify the means.

Some of the worst social atrocities (e.g., slavery) and medical horrors (e.g., fatal experiments on subjects without their consent) have been the result of this way of thinking. Sometimes the number of people negatively affected by a practice is so high that it is difficult to get the calculations of overall benefit to justify the practice. In such cases, there is a great temptation to consider those who will be harmed as less than fully human so that the impact on them will not have to receive full weight. Sometimes this is done blatantly, as when the U.S. Constitutional Convention considered a slave to be "three-fifths of a person" for certain purposes. More often it is done subtly when the decision makers determine how much weight to attach to the negative consequences affecting certain people.

These problems have understandably convinced many that a bioethics of consequences is mistaken. They recognize that certain things are wrong, regardless of who benefits how much from them, and so they champion instead a bioethics of *principles*. An ethics of principles holds that there are one or more principles that must be observed in any situation before any other considerations are ethically relevant. Examples of such principles include a mandate to uphold freedom, justice, and life.

An ethics of principles holds that there are one or more principles that must be observed in any situation before any other considerations are ethically relevant.

The very idea of principles is appealing because it agrees with our sense that everything is not up for grabs ethically, depending on the circumstances. There are definite rights and wrongs. This approach also has the appeal of avoiding all of the workability problems attached to a bioethics of consequences. Particularly attractive among the principles is the principle of freedom—or "autonomy" as it is sometimes called—since it insures that people will be given the responsibility to make the decisions that most seriously affect their own lives. In fact, this principle is so important for many that they consider it to be the only absolute principle.

However, a bioethics of principles, in any form, has its own serious problems. How do we know which principles are valid? Every person in a situation may affirm a different set of principles. Moreover, how are conflicts between principles to be resolved? Everyone may have a different set of priorities. It all comes down to one person's intuition versus another's, and the opportunities for biased and self-serving bioethics are unending.

This is particularly the case when the principle of freedom, or autonomy, receives exclusive focus. The word *autonomy* comes from two Greek words meaning "self law." In other words, in this approach to bioethics, the self becomes its own ethical law. Whatever the self decides, is right for that person. The well-being of others need not be considered. In theory, people are to respect the autonomy of others, but those focused on their own autonomy—self-centered beings that we are—are not likely to be as concerned about the well-being of others as they are about their own.

Despite the great influence of this way of thinking in society today, especially in matters of bioethics, we have not yet experienced anything like the most negative impact it can have. The biblical values embedded in Judeo-Christian culture have fostered an intuitive regard for others in most people. But as these influences in public education and other public arenas continue to diminish—in the name of pluralism, including separation of church and state—the self-centeredness of autonomy ethics will become more apparent. The risk to others is real.

Here is where the danger of this approach begins to resemble that of a bioethics of consequences. As long as people are similarly prominent and powerful, protecting their freedom to pursue their own benefit is fine. However, those who are weaker physically, socially, or economically may not be able to do so very effectively. And where the principle of autonomy rules, there are no other equally strong ethical norms such as justice or love to safeguard those unable to promote their own interests and welfare.

Some people, taking the deficiencies of human nature quite seriously, reject both a bioethics of consequences and a bioethics of principles. They are concerned that both offer a way to identify the right thing to do but pay no attention to the person who must do it. What good is it, they observe, for people to identify what is right if they lack the character to do it?

Because of the great importance of this observation, it is worthwhile to say a few things about the alternative that these critics propose, even though the number of people who advocate this alternative today is far smaller than the number who support the other two approaches. These critics advocate instead a bioethics of *virtues*. The essence of this approach is that ethics should focus on helping people to develop good character traits or virtues, and that right actions will flow from good character.

Good character can make a significant difference in how both in-

> **T**he essence of a bioethics of virtues is that ethics should focus on helping people to develop good character traits or virtues, and that right actions will flow from good character.

dividual and social bioethical challenges are handled. Virtuous physicians and patients' family members who are genuinely committed to the well-being of mentally disabled patients are more likely than those less virtuous to make the best end-of-life treatment decisions for such patients. Similarly, virtuous health care administrators who are sensitive to the needs of all types of patients are more likely than those less virtuous to make the best resource allocation decisions.

As necessary as virtues are if people are to live as they should in the face of challenges to life and health, however, this alternative approach to bioethics has some serious deficiencies. Have you ever been in a situation where you honestly felt that you had the right attitude ethically—that you truly wanted to do the right thing in the eyes of all—but you simply didn't know what that was? That's not an unusual experience. Regardless of how virtuous people are in general or in a particular situation, they still need some way to recognize the right thing to do. Being virtuous makes us willing to do what is right, but it doesn't always tell us how to identify what is right.

Even if right decisions always flowed straight from good character, there would be some difficulties analogous to those discussed above concerning a bioethics of principles. For instance, which virtues should we cultivate? The virtues promoted by the philosopher Aristotle are not the same as those espoused by the theologian Dietrich Bonhoeffer. Moreover, our fallen human natures render us necessarily self-centered, and selfishness is one of the great enemies of virtue. On the basis of our own desires and ability, how virtuous can we be expected to become?

Where does all this leave us? Contemporary bioethics provides helpful tools for understanding and addressing ethical conflicts. It also offers various forms of reasoning to enable us to engage bioethical challenges. However, each form of reasoning is quite inadequate, for the reasons noted. That observation compels us, and other thinking people, to take an honest look at what a biblical approach has to offer. As the next chapter explains, a biblical approach to bioethics is justified in making the amazing claim that it avoids the problems of the other approaches and yet retains their strengths.

3 Does the Bible Address Bioethics?

While many Christians automatically look to the Bible to guide them in their daily lives, they may not think to look there for counsel on the new bioethical issues of today. Non-Christians may assume that the ethical guidance to be found there is less useful than the worldly wisdom they can find elsewhere. Both groups are in for a surprise: Christians because of the Bible's relevance; non-Christians because the Bible avoids all of the ethical shortcomings of other contemporary approaches to bioethics discussed in the previous chapter.

The Bible speaks to bioethics, though not by explicitly calling the issues by name: cloning, stem cell research, and so forth. Any book of such counsel would be out of date soon after it was written. Rather, it offers something much more valuable, more timeless, more applicable to newly-emerging issues. It provides a way of looking at the world—a way of thinking—that enables us to grapple with the toughest issues of life. While this way of thinking can be described in many different ways, three of its most central characteristics are that it is God-centered, reality-bounded, and love-impelled.

A God-Centered Bioethics

To say that bioethics, from a biblical perspective, should be God-centered is to suggest two things: that human reason alone is inadequate and that God is more than adequate. The problem with a human-centered bioethics, one depending solely on reason, is that people are sinful. The human race was created to follow God's ways, knowing and trusting that flourishing would result.

However, as Genesis 3 tells the story, people decided to adopt their own standards rather than God's, and they became preoccupied with themselves as a result. That is what sin is about—our focus on self rather than on God and others. Since we are so preoccupied, or sinful, we have lost the ability to do what is good consistently. Accordingly, the Old and New Testaments alike observe that "all have turned away; . . . there is no one who does good" (Romans 3:12; see also Psalm 14:3).

The point is not that people never do particular things that are good. Rather, they lack the intimate connection with God that would enable their reason to recognize consistently what is good, as opposed to what is merely self-serving. There is a built-in resistance to live as God has designed us to live, whether conscious or unconscious: "The sinful mind is hostile to God. It does not submit to God's law, nor can it do so" (Romans 8:7).

So a biblical bioethics challenges us to recognize that we cannot live as we ought unless we are willing to look to God to provide a standard for our character and direction for our thinking. God knows everything and so is able to take everyone and everything into consideration in a way that we cannot. Moreover, God is good, modeling a perfect blend of truthfulness and compassion, of justice and mercy. God's Spirit is a Holy Spirit, who cultivates in us a character that is holy (set apart from the world) and righteous (in line with God's standards). The virtues

> **A** biblical bioethics challenges us to recognize that we cannot live as we ought unless we are willing to look to God to provide a standard for our character and direction for our thinking.

of character are seen in the fruit of the Spirit: "love, joy, peace, patience, kindness, goodness, faithfulness, gentleness and self-control" (Galatians 5:22-23; cf. 1 Thessalonians 4:7-8). Such character enables us to recognize and do what is right, with God's ongoing direction. God is continually renewing the minds of those who look to him for guidance, so that they "will be able to test and approve what God's will is—his good, pleasing and perfect will" (Romans 12:2).

To make all this more concretely visible to us, God took on human form in the person of Jesus Christ. In Jesus we get a clear picture of who God is: "The Son is the radiance of God's glory and the exact representation of his being, sustaining all things by his powerful word" (Hebrews 1:3). We see the perfect image of God, for example, protecting the weak—those without voice in the world. So we, too, created in God's image, are to stand up for the powerless (see Colossians 3:12-13), whether they are racial minorities receiving inadequate access to health care or embryonic human beings destroyed in order to develop stem cell treatments for the rest of us. As Jesus put it, the important question is not, "Who is my neighbor" and worthy of my love? but rather, Am I a neighbor and loving as a neighbor should love (see Luke 10:29-37)?

This God-centered orientation has major implications for how we respond to the bioethical challenges of our day. We will not see fetuses as dispensable because they are weak and voiceless. Rather, we will defend the defenseless. But if we are truly to *be* a neighbor rather than remain preoccupied with who should be included in the human community, we will be just as concerned about how we can support the mother who does not know how she can possibly go through with her pregnancy.

Similarly, we will not kill (or assist the killing) of older patients who despair of continuing to live. In the Incarnation, God became one of us, enduring our suffering and bearing our burdens. If we are to exhibit true compassion—literally "suffering with"—we, too, will be incarnational and do all we can to bear the burdens of dying patients with them. We will not get rid of the problems by getting rid of the patients.

Being God-centered in our approach to bioethics is an important starting point. But that is just the beginning of a biblical bioethics.

A Reality-Bounded Bioethics

God also directs us in his written word to be realistic! Being realistic means understanding reality— the way things really are—and living in accordance with it. We do this all the time in everyday life. If the bridge over a raging river has been washed away and we need to take a fifteen-minute detour to the next bridge, we are "realistic" if we allow fifteen extra minutes to get to our destination across the river. If we think that we can fly our car across the river, and attempt to do so, we are more than unrealistic—we are destructive. A man may say, "The idea that the bridge is missing may be part of your reality, but it's not part of mine!" But if we follow his lead, we are foolish.

The Bible affirms the importance of living realistically—according to the way things really are—but it also reminds us that there is more to reality than what we perceive with our physical senses. God has made the world and everything in it in a certain way. To flourish, we need to know what that reality looks like and to make sure that we live in accordance with it.

If we are playing a ball game in a small field on the edge of a cliff, we could say that freedom and happiness mean simply running wherever we want to, paying no attention to where we are running. That would be foolish, though, because it would be unrealistic. We would either be injured running off the cliff, or we would be seriously inhibited by the need to constantly assess how close we were to the cliff in order to avoid injury. If someone put up a fence a safe distance from the cliff, we could claim that it stifled our freedom and happiness, but we would be mistaken. Only with such a fence in place could we play free from preoccupation and injury.

God alone can see all of the reality that exists. But in the Bible he describes for us much of what is beyond the reach of our limited physical senses, so that with "eyes of faith" we can see it too. So that we don't miss the point of that description, God shows us not only the cliffs but also the fences we must realistically live within if we are to live with freedom and happiness. He also reminds us not to focus *too* much on the fences and cliffs, for if we look the other way, we will see the open lands on which God intends us to prosper.

What are some examples of these humanly invisible aspects of reality that God alerts us to in the Bible? Some are in the past, some in the present, and others in the future. Past aspects of reality with implications for how we should live include the facts that it was God who created the world itself (Psalm 89) and that Jesus Christ's death paid the penalty for our sins (see Romans 6). Present aspects include the fact that every human being, though fallen, is created in the image of God (see Genesis 9:6; James 3:9). Future aspects of reality include the certainty of Christ's return to judge everyone (see 1 Thessalonians 4:13–5:11).

Sometimes biblical writers draw direct ethical conclusions from such aspects of reality. However, sometimes there is an intermediate step: identifying and describing the fences that signal an important reality is close at hand. For example, human beings have a special status in the biblical writings, and much ethical instruction is devoted to ways that *human life* (meaning human beings) should be respected and protected. The reason for such a high regard is the reality that human beings are created in the image of God. Ethical guidance, though, may simply refer to what should be done in support of human life—that is, refrain from murder (see Exodus 20:13) or build cities of refuge (see Deuteronomy 19:5-7). Nevertheless, the implicit basis of life's importance is its place in the reality of how God has created and intended the world to be.

The implications of this reality alone in the realm of bioethics are huge. If we are to avoid destroying something as important as human life, then how much more the killing of patients (by themselves or others) is wrong. We must also avoid endangering the lives of anything that could well be a human being. So we must devote serious attention to the question of whether or not fetuses or embryos are human beings. If they are, then we must be very careful about how we handle them. Certain reproductive technologies, for instance, may not be inherently unethical; but some ways of using them endanger human embryos in a way that others do not, and those uses would need to be avoided.

There are more biblical fences, though, than life. *Justice* is another particularly important fence. Because of the reality that all people are created in the image of God, their lives are equally significant (similar cases should be treated similarly), and a life-threatening need warrants special effort to meet that need. This is called justice in the biblical writings (see Jeremiah 22:15-16; 2 Corinthians 8:13-15). Justice has crucial implications for resource allocation questions, among other issues. Not only does it call for adequate resources to be devoted to health care, it also insists that certain types of people not be unfairly discriminated against when they need vital treatments. Unjust discrimination is an emerging problem in the genetics arena as well. People are increasingly at risk of being unjustly denied jobs or other benefits on the basis of genetic information that predicts the mere possibility of health problems.

A third example of a biblical fence is *freedom*. People are created and intended by God to be free, in the basic sense of free from a variety of oppressive conditions such as slavery (see Jeremiah 34:17; 1 Corinthians 7:21-23; Philemon 1:14-16). But freedom is not just an end in itself; it is also a means to a greater end. People are freed for something and not merely from something. Freedom is a state of doing as much as it is a state of being (see Galatians 5:1; James 1:25). People are freed to live the God-centered, reality-bounded, love-impelled life being described here.

So people are free, for example, to decide whether or not they want life-sustaining treatments when they are dying. It is not appropriate for others to force treatment on them. However, freedom in this sense does not mean that whatever treatment decisions people make are the right ones, simply because they are what people want. Such an idea would be the contemporary notion of "autonomy" criticized in the previous chapter. Freedom is rightly exercised in support of life and everything else that God deems important, not exercised in a way that intentionally fosters death by leaving a treatable condition untreated.

A Love-Impelled Bioethics

This mention of freedom reminds us that a biblical approach to bioethics is not nearly as constraining as we might think if we focused too long on the ways that the realities of the world limit how we should live. There are, indeed, some limits. But in so many situations, few or none of the options before us are ruled out by such reality-bounded considerations as being life-threatening, unjust, and so on. In cases where more than one option is within the limits, how do we decide which option is best? One word: love.

We are to "follow the way of love," for it is "the most excellent way" (1 Corinthians 14:1; 12:31). It is what the various commandments detailing our obligations to our neighbors are all about (see Romans 13:8-9; Galatians 5:14). To love is to do that which will enable people to experience as much "good" as possible, that they might be built up (see 1 Corinthians 8:1; 10:24). Jesus illustrates such love of neighbor in very concrete terms: the Good Samaritan meeting the life and health needs of the man beaten half dead on the road to Jericho (see Luke 10:29-37).

Freedom is rightly exercised in support of life and everything else that God deems important, not exercised in a way that intentionally fosters death by leaving a treatable condition untreated.

On another occasion, Jesus elaborates on the place of loving our neighbor in the larger scheme of things (Matthew 22:34-40). His instruction comes in response to a question as to which of all the commandments is the greatest. The first and greatest, Jesus says, is the command to love God. But "the second is like it: 'Love your neighbor as yourself.' " Furthermore, he observes, it is these two commands together that are the essence of what the Bible ("the Law and the Prophets") requires. In other words, our first responsibility is to love God, which in ethical terms means to follow a God-centered and reality-bounded ethics—living in accordance with how God has created and intended the world to be. Then, within those bounds, our next responsibility is to love our neighbor as ourself, which in ethical terms is the love-impelled ethics that seeks human well-being.

Even loving our neighbors, though, is to be patterned after God's own love. As God is actively involved in sustaining those in need, so God's people are to be actively involved (see, for example, Isaiah 25:4; 58:6-7). In the New Testament, the pattern becomes specifically Christ-centered. In the words of Jesus, "As I have loved you, so you must love one another" (John 13:34; 15:12). Jesus shows us what love looks like in the face of sickness and other needs (Matthew 4:23-24; Luke 4:18-19) and calls us to live in the same way (Mark 16:18; Luke 16:19-31). If we do not follow the example of Jesus' self-sacrifice in tangible, day-to-day ways, then God's love is not in us. "We know what real love is because Christ gave up his life for us. And so we also ought to give up our lives for our Christian brothers and sisters. But if anyone has enough money to live well and sees a brother or sister in need and refuses to help—how can God's love be in that person?" (1 John 3:16-27, NLT)

While love does require particular actions, it involves more than that. Even actions beneficial to others but done with the wrong motive will receive no recognition (or no "credit") from God. "If I give . . . but have not love, I gain nothing" (1 Corinthians 13:3). Intention matters. Love is not merely an externally imposed standard; it is an inwardly motivating virtue of Spirit-filled persons (Galatians 5:22-23). God wants more than people who give to others out of mere compulsion: "God loves a cheerful giver" (2 Corinthians 9:7).

So a biblical bioethics involves far more than simply applying a specific set of God-given rules. There are indeed many aspects of reality that have implications for right and wrong living. But recognizing which ones apply in a given situation requires discernment. Then, once we have excluded ethically unacceptable ways of approaching that situation, love requires a careful assessment of the remaining alternatives. We must judge, for each alternative, how people will be affected if we pursue it. We need the best counsel possible to help us recognize what love beckons us to do. That means, most importantly, that we must seek direction from God in prayer (see Psalm 16:7). God often provides the wisdom we seek through the counsel of people, so we should also seek out and be open to such counsel: "The way of a fool seems right to him, but a wise man listens to advice" (Proverbs 12:15; cf. 2 Corinthians 8:21). We particularly need to seek counsel from those who are experienced in loving God and their neighbors.

A love-impelled approach has major implications for every issue in bioethics. For example, if a patient is in the final days of a dying process, it is acceptable to decide against attempting a treatment that will probably add burden to the dying process without significantly extending the patient's life. No God-given realities are violated by doing so. However, that does not mean that it is necessarily right to withhold the treatment. Whether or not to withhold it depends on a love-impelled consideration of what will benefit the patient the most, all things considered. The burden of the treatment, the opportunity to communicate meaningfully with others, and various other factors must be weighed. Similarly, there may be nothing inherently wrong with certain

> **W**e particularly need to seek counsel from those who are experienced in loving God and their neighbors.

reproductive, genetic, or other emerging technologies. In other words, there may be uses for them that do not conflict with how God has created and intended the world to be. Nevertheless, whether it is ethical to use them in a particular situation will depend on how people will be helped or hurt by them.

A Biblical Example

As we have noted, many of today's life and health issues are not explicitly mentioned in the Bible. But that does not mean the Bible is irrelevant to bioethics. To the contrary, the Bible offers something much more valuable, more timeless, more applicable to newly emerging issues than a time-bound set of prescriptions. It provides a way of looking at the world—a way of thinking—that enables us to grapple with the toughest issues of life. Nevertheless, it is helpful to look at how the Bible explicitly wrestles with specific issues in order to clarify how this way of thinking applies in practice. One such issue in biblical times was male circumcision. Examining how Paul decided when this surgical procedure was right to do and when it was not will help illustrate how the biblical approach described above works in practice.

To take a position on this issue, Paul first has to consider what God's view of it is. Does God either require or forbid all men to be circumcised? Paul knows that if either is the case, it is because some reality-bounded consideration is at stake. Either circumcision would be a necessary part of—or would violate—how God has created male human beings to be. In the former case, circumcision would be required in every situation; in the latter, it would always be forbidden. Paul concludes, however, that "circumcision is nothing and uncircumcision is nothing" (1 Corinthians 7:19).

That means the right answer to the circumcision question will be sensitive to the context. A discerning love-impelled decision will be required. So when a question arises about circumcising Titus in Galatia, Paul says circumcision would be wrong. To give in to the demands of some people there to circumcise Titus would be to agree that for Titus to become a true believer, he needed to follow all the ceremonial requirements of Jewish law. That would mean people would have to try to earn their way to God by following a set of rules. As a result, they would miss the gospel message that eternal life with God comes through faith, not by works, and countless numbers of people would never know God. Love for his neighbors required Paul to oppose Titus's circumcision (see Galatians 2:1-6, 14-16).

In Lystra, however, Paul encountered a very different situation involving Timothy. Timothy's lack of circumcision in that predominantly Jewish area was both known and offensive to people there. The problem was more a Jewish cultural one than a theological or ethical issue of the sort Paul confronted in Galatia. The people intuitively reacted negatively to men who were uncircumcised, perhaps somewhat like the way some people today react to men with earrings in their noses and ears. Because they wouldn't take such a man seriously, many who otherwise would hear the gospel message and come to know God through Timothy would not do so unless Timothy was circumcised. So love for his neighbors required Paul to support Timothy's circumcision (see Acts 16:1-5).

How Biblical and Other Approaches Compare

To see just how distinctive and attractive this biblical approach to bioethics is, let's compare it with the three other popular but flawed approaches discussed in chapter 2. We will find that each of these three approaches takes a part of the biblical approach and makes it the whole. That explains why each is so appealing to so many people: Each affirms something that is in line with how God has intended things to be. It also explains why each is so problematic: Each leaves out multiple God-intended provisions that otherwise would guard each approach from its worst deficiencies.

Take, for example, a bioethics of consequences. It is so preoccupied with the love-impelled dimension of a biblical bioethics that it makes it the whole of bioethics. Seeking the well-being of people is indeed extremely important. But when the love-impelled dimension is pulled out of the biblical framework, the other two tiers of the framework are lost. Love of neighbor becomes more important than love of God—which is backward. Lacking a God-centered dimension, a bioethics of consequences typically pays no attention to the importance of character in bioethics. Even its assessment of consequences tends to be faulty, since it typically overlooks spiritual and eternal consequences.

At the same time, without a reality-bounded dimension, it is extremely risky. It disregards parts of reality and says we can do whatever we want, as long as people receive enough benefit. Those who play by its rules are like the ballplayers in the field at the edge of the cliff without fences. Much of the time the actual playing is fine. But eventually people will be seriously injured falling off the cliff, since the game is being played as if the cliff were not there. A bioethics of consequences is similarly bound to produce oppressive and destructive results periodically, as discussed in chapter 2. For example, it may justify denying vital health care resources to those considered least valuable to society. Or it may advocate sacrificing a limited number of the youngest among us in experiments to develop cloning technologies and stem cell treatments for the benefit of many.

A bioethics of principles has the same sort of weaknesses. It is so enamored of one part of biblical bioethics—in this case the reality-bounded dimension—that it makes it the whole of bioethics. Its appeal is that it affirms that there are certain rights and wrongs in life, that is, principles. However, without a God-centered dimension, it lacks the single and sure basis that a biblical bioethics provides for right and wrong and for the character people need in order to live out what they identify is right. In fact, without God, even the reality-bounded dimension of this approach is faulty. People need the mind of Christ—"be transformed by the renewing of your mind" (Romans 12:2) and "have the mind of Christ" (1 Corinthians 2:16)—in order to perceive reality accurately and identify and prioritize the right principles.

Without a love-impelled dimension, a bioethics of principles operates under the illusion that there is a principle or rule for everything. It can easily degenerate into a loveless legalism. Of course, it may try to compensate by making concern for human well-being one of its principles. However, such concern is then likely to override other basic principles at times, creating the problems of a bioethics of consequences just noted.

A bioethics of virtues has similar drawbacks. It takes part of the God-centered dimension of bioethics, the importance of character, and makes it the whole. Its recognition of character explains its appeal. But as discussed previously, God and God's written Word are essential if we are to have a single and sure standard for what the virtues are that make up good character. Moreover, without the Spirit of Christ alive within us, we cannot be the virtuous people we would like to be.

Meanwhile, the other two dimensions of a biblical bioethics are left out entirely. Concretely, that means we lack any way to identify what the right thing to do is in a complex situation, no matter how willing we are to do it because of our virtuous character. For instance, we may fail to recognize some crucially relevant aspect of reality—such as the missing bridge over a raging river—and inadvertently cause great harm. That is how well-intentioned people can end up supporting unethical practices such as assisted suicide and unlimited genetic designing of human beings. They intend good, but they do not consider everything that is ethically relevant in order to identify what the good is.

Recognizing the similarities and differences between a biblical bioethics and other popular approaches to bioethics can be helpful for several reasons. It helps us understand why other approaches to bioethics are so intuitively appealing to many: They contain an element of truth. And while this is not enough to make good decisions, it does show us where to look for common ground with people who do not affirm a biblical bioethics when we are building coalitions to address bioethical issues in public policy. And it alerts us to the major shortcomings of other approaches when common ground on a bioethical issue is not possible and we need to explain why a biblical approach is the wisest course to follow.

PART TWO

□ □ □ □ □

HEALTH CARE:
Across the Lifespan

4 Embryonic Ethics: Stem Cell Research, Abortion, and Beyond

Many of the most challenging bioethical issues in health care arise at the beginning of life. Some of the issues center on the kinds of research that are acceptable in order to develop new medical treatments. Other issues have to do with the kinds of medical procedures that are acceptable in order to benefit patients. One example of the first type is stem cell research; an example of the second is abortion.

Stem Cell Research

Because stem cell research is so controversial today, many people mistakenly think it is something that is either good or bad—something you are for or against. But that is far from the case. Stem cell research has multiple forms that raise very different ethical issues.

Stem cells take their name from the stem of a plant. The various parts of a plant—branches, leaves, and flowers—all originate from the stem. Similarly, in humans a stem cell is a type of cell from which many other more specialized cells develop—for example, blood cells, nerve cells, and muscle cells.

Although stem cells can be classified in many ways, there are three types of stem cells whose differences are especially significant ethically: adult, fetal, and embryonic. *Adult stem cells* are cells that can be taken from any human being who has already been born (not just adults), without harming that person. These stem cells are found in human blood, bone marrow, skin, brain tissue, and other parts of the body, including the placenta and umbilical cord that connect baby and mother.

On the other hand, *fetal stem cells* are typically taken from a fetus's bone marrow or sex-related cells (which will develop into ovaries in females or testes in males). They are most often taken from aborted fetuses, but they can also come from miscarried or stillborn fetuses, or potentially from fetuses still alive in the womb. *Embryonic stem cells* come from embryos approximately 7 to 10 days old. The embryonic period lasts from fertilization (when the man's sperm and woman's egg join—or the equivalent of this in the cloning process—see chapter 8) until the embryo becomes a fetus approximately 7 weeks later. The embryo is destroyed in the process of harvesting embryonic stem cells.

The great appeal of stem cell research is that there is ample evidence it will lead to cures or improved treatments for many medical conditions such as diabetes and strokes. Already, patients suffering from sickle-cell anemia, multiple sclerosis, and heart damage have been significantly helped by treatments involving adult stem cells. Stem cells should also provide a way to grow tissues and organs in the lab, which can save the lives of many patients such as those dying from Parkinson's Disease or liver failure. Since adult stem cells can be obtained without risk to the donor, these wonderful benefits should be wholeheartedly supported by everyone.

> **The great appeal of stem cell research is that there is ample evidence it will lead to cures or improved treatments for many medical conditions.**

Ethical problems arise only when the donor is seriously harmed in the process. Such is always the case with embryonic stem cells, so the difference between adult and embryonic cells will provide a useful focus for our ethical analysis here.

However, the donor may also be seriously harmed in the case of fetal stem cells, so we will return to them at the end of this chapter.

How serious is it to kill a human embryo, ethically speaking? The answer depends on whether or not an embryo is a human being who should be protected from harm just like any other human being. If we would at least go so far as to say that human embryos have *some* value, then they should not be harmed if doing so can be avoided. In terms of the stem cell debate, that would mean stem cell research that kills embryos is wrong if the benefits of stem cell research can be obtained another way, without such killing.

It turns out that there does appear to be another way: adult stem cell research. To date, adult stem cell research has led to a large number of successful medical treatments, as described above, and tens of thousands of adult stem cell therapies are carried out each year in the U.S. alone. On the other hand, embryonic stem cells have actually produced relatively few medical benefits in patients and are rarely being employed in treatments.

In fact, using embryonic rather than adult cells makes it more likely that harmful tumors will develop. Because embryonic cells are less focused than adult cells, they are more likely to cause unwanted growth along with desired growth. A further advantage of adult cells is that when patients are treated using cells from their own bodies, their bodies are less likely to reject them than if the treatment involves embryonic cells containing a genetic code different from their own.

Since the use of adult stem cells has such advantages, it may seem surprising that embryonic stem cell research is even being pursued. The main driving force has been the theory that embryonic stem cells may ultimately prove to be more useful than adult cells because they may be more flexible. Adult stem cells have already specialized into particular types of stem cells—blood stem cells to produce blood, muscle stem cells to produce muscle, and so on. Embryonic stem cells have not yet specialized at all: they have the potential to produce any of the 210 kinds of material in the human body. Fetal stem cells are somewhere in between—more specialized than embryonic cells but less so than adult cells.

However, recent research now suggests that adult stem cells can be extremely flexible as well. One study has found that certain cells in the bone marrow of adults can probably produce any type of cell in the body. Another has found stem cells in the blood of adults so flexible that they can produce tissue for vital organs, such as the liver.[1] So it is becoming increasingly apparent that embryonic stem cell research will not be necessary in order to achieve the desired medical results. Therefore, if there is anything undesirable about harming human embryos, then only adult stem cell research should be pursued. By no means should human embryos be created for the purpose of embryonic stem cell research.

Nevertheless, there are those who find the status of human embryos to be hopelessly unclear. As a result, just the possibility that some unexpected useful discovery could come from embryonic stem cell research is enough to justify the freedom to pursue it in their eyes. If there were sufficient reason to consider the human embryo to be a human being worthy of the same protections given any other human being, that would be a different story. So before this chapter concludes, we will take a closer look at the question of who is a human being. (We will use the term "human being," since "human life" as popularly used can mean merely living human tissue, such as skin; and "person" is a legal term which can mean something slightly different than its ethical counterpart, "human being.")

Abortion and Beyond

Before turning to the question of whether or not an embryo (not to mention a fetus) is a human being, it is important to note that many other bioethical issues hinge on this question. The most familiar of these is the abortion issue, since a decision to abort necessarily involves the death of an embryo or fetus. To date, many in the abortion debate have attempted to sidestep this question by claiming that a woman's right to control her body outweighs the importance of the life in the womb. But on closer examination, this claim is usually tied to the view that the life in the womb is not really a human being in the fullest sense. For most people recognize that the right to life is more basic than rights concerning what we can or cannot do while we are alive.

Nevertheless, this evasion will become irrelevant in the next decade or so when the artificial womb is perfected. Its development is already well along. When it becomes available and a woman wants to exercise her right to control her body by ending her pregnancy, doing so will no longer require killing a fetus. Instead, an artificial womb will be able to sustain the fetus until a womb is no longer required to keep the child alive. In fact, if the fetus is recognized to be a human being or to have special significance for some other reason, killing the fetus will be considered unethical because a mechanical womb is available to complete the pregnancy. So clarity regarding the status of human embryos and fetuses will be essential.

There are many other bioethical issues where such clarity is essential as well. Many of the reproductive methods discussed in chapter 7 as well as cloning issues discussed in chapter 8 involve dangers to the embryo. The ever-improving capability to diagnose genetic problems in embryos and fetuses discussed in chapter 9 creates temptations to eliminate ones that are not quite what we wanted.

So many important bioethical issues hinge on the question of whether or not human embryos (and therefore fetuses as well) are human beings who should be treated as such. We cannot avoid answering this question if we want to reach ethical conclusions on these issues. If we allow (even if we do not favor) any action that involves killing embryos, then we have in fact answered the question—we have not avoided it. We have answered that we are confident the embryo is not a human being. A careful review of the scientific and scriptural evidence reveals that such confidence is not warranted.

What Science Tells Us about Embryos

Increasingly, people are coming to recognize that even the earliest embryo is not just a blob of material. Rather, that embryo is a highly sophisticated entity in which each cell, starting at the single cell stage, contains a genetic code of instructions involving 3 billion pairs of chemicals. This code has been compared to a code of 3 billion letters. Since there are six letters in the average word, this code could be compared to 500 million words. With about 300 words on a printed page and 250 pages in a book, the human genetic code would make up 8,000 books—with copies contained within each cell of the human embryo from the earliest

> **The embryo is a highly sophisticated entity in which each cell, starting at the single cell stage, contains a genetic code of instructions involving 3 billion pairs of chemicals.**

stage, actively directing the growth of a human being.[2]

Admittedly, the human embryo doesn't look like you do now. But that embryo is exactly what you looked like at that stage in your development. From the very beginning of our lives, at the first cell stage, the code and the life were in place to direct everything. All that was needed was a hospitable environment (at first a womb, then a setting with air and shelter) and the provision of raw materials (some combination of liquid/water and nutrients/food) so that our genetically-guided bodies could use those materials to build and re-build our bodies in various ways. A self-developing living entity, a full human genetic code, a suitable environment with suitable nurture—that, biologically describes a living human adult. That also, biologically, is a living human embryo. Both alike are human beings.

We should be candid and admit that this conclusion is something we may resist, as many others resist it, because it is so inconvenient. It would be far easier if the embryo could be dismissed as just some blob of material. We would then be free to do whatever we want with it, for our benefit.

But we could label any group of people "sub-human" in order to justify the pursuit of our own benefit at their expense. In fact, we have done so in the past, with African-American slaves. Even the U.S. Supreme Court in the Dred Scott case identified them as mere property, rather than persons with full human rights, in order to justify denying to them the protections normally due to any human being.

It seems so obvious to us now how blinded people were by perhaps unthinkingly adopting an ethics of consequences (see chapter 2). The benefit to be gained by those in control seemed so great, and the people in view looked so different from the rest that it was all too easy not to consider them persons.

But we must consider how *we* will look, generations from now. Will people look back on all of the genetic data that is becoming widely known today and shake their heads as we do over those in the Dred Scott generation? Sadly, they did not give honest consideration to the personhood of American slaves because of the benefits they would have to give up if black people could not be used for the "greater good." How about us, regarding the embryo?

When the assumption that the embryo is not a person is driven by personal convenience and preference and not by science, people may be convicted at this point. But some will insist that there is a meaningful scientific difference between an embryo and an adult human being. They will suggest some characteristic, possessed by adults but not by embryos, which is essential to have before one is a human being. If there is such a characteristic, then there would be a legitimate reason not to view an embryo as a human being. So let's consider here the primary alternatives for when, after fertilization, a human being first comes into existence—from the latest to the earliest.

- Some will say that there is no human being until *sometime during infancy,* since that is the first point at which there is self-consciousness. But adults can lose consciousness—not to mention self-consciousness—and we don't say they are no longer human beings.

- Others will say that we have a human being *once birth takes place,* since at that point the baby is no longer connected to and totally dependent on something or someone else.

But adults can become connected to and totally dependent on a ventilator to breathe for them in the same way—and we don't say they are no longer human beings.

☐ Still others will say that we become human beings *before birth, at the point of viability,* since that by definition is when the fetus is capable of living independently should birth take place. But conjoined twins or adults dependent on pacemakers are not capable of living independently in that way— yet we don't say they are not human beings.

☐ Many have said that a human being is present at the point *when the fetus shows movement,* traditionally measured by when the mother feels the fetus move. But adults can become paralyzed, and we don't say they are no longer human beings.

☐ More recently, some have said that we have a human being about six weeks after fertilization, *when brain activity is detectable,* since that is when the potential for self-consciousness is present. But when adults lose consciousness, they can also lose the potential for self-consciousness—yet we don't say they are no longer human beings.

☐ Even more recently, others have begun saying that a human being is first present *when the embryo attaches to the wall of a mother's uterus* (the point of *implantation*), since without that attachment the embryo cannot live. But when adults lose the capacity to breathe on their own and are in desperate need of being attached to a ventilator in order to live, we don't say they are no longer human beings until they are attached.

In other words, there is no point later than fertilization after which an embryo, fetus, or child gains something that an adult has, which is essential in order to be a human being. There is no capability or potential that makes something more definitively a human being than what genetics has already established at fertilization.

What Scripture Tells Us about Embryos

Christians will also be interested in what the Bible has to say on such matters. But it has been important to establish first that the issue of when a human being begins to exist is not simply a religious matter. The best science and logic point in the same direction as Scripture.

As discussed in chapter 3, biblically sound bioethics is centered in God and rooted in reality—in how God has made the

There is no capability or potential that makes something more definitively a human being than what genetics has already established at fertilization.

world and what God has done in history. In order to understand who the embryo is, we more specifically need to consider the implications of how God has created human beings and how God has intervened to restore them. For if God has identified with human life not simply in its adult form but even at the embryonic stage, then all of the protections due to human beings apply to embryos as well as adults.

The first way God identifies with human beings is by creating them in his very own image. In Genesis 1:26-27 we read about the initial creation of the human race in God's image: "Then God said, 'Let us make man in our image, in our likeness. . . . So God created man in his own image, in the image of God he created him; male and female he created them." Genesis 9:6 later makes it clear that all human beings are created in God's image, and that a human life is therefore not to be taken unjustly.

For if God has identified with human life not simply in its adult form but even at the embryonic stage, then all of the protections due to human beings apply to embryos as well as adults.

Killing an innocent human being warrants the worst possible punishment, explains God, precisely because people are created in his image: "Whoever sheds the blood of man, by man shall his blood be shed; for in the image of God has God made man" (Genesis 9:6).

What is it, then, to which the image of God is attached? Most importantly, it is not a definitive set of characteristics or abilities or functions of people that warrant this connection with God—that make it appropriate to label their creation as "in God's image." Rather, Scripture simply affirms: that which is alive and human is in God's image. The contrast in Genesis 1 is explicitly between human beings and all other living things. The fact that life is human rather than non-human is what identifies it as in the image of God. We know today that this distinction is present at the earliest, single-cell stage, when the genetics of the embryo already distinguish this life as human, as opposed to something other than human. Because people are created in God's image, there are certain God-like characteristics that people typically have, including various mental, moral, spiritual, and relational capacities. But being created in God's image does not depend on having any particular one of those characteristics.

Scientific and scriptural evidence together—both genetics and Genesis—point to divine involvement in the creation of human beings even at the embryonic stage. And because human embryos are created in God's image, various passages of Scripture affirm and reflect on the preciousness of human life in the womb.

Psalm 139, for instance, opens with six verses on the vastness of God: God knows everything and is everywhere. The next six verses describe our natural bent to try to escape from God—to find some situation in which we can do with our life whatever we want.

Scientific and scriptural evidence together—both genetics and Genesis—point to divine involvement in the creation of human beings even at the embryonic stage.

The psalmist then points out that there is no such place to avoid God even in the womb—even at the stage when there is an "unformed body" (an apt description of the embryo). Even in the womb nothing is hidden from God. When we do something "in the womb" (i.e., to the embryo), we are not in some realm of "private choice" or science in which we are welcome to do with an unborn human being whatever we think will benefit us. The embryo is created in the very image of God, and God is watching in the womb (not to mention in the more visible lab) to see how we are treating that image.

As previously noted, God also has another major connection with the embryo. It is through the Incarnation, when God became a human being, Jesus Christ. If only adults are human beings, or one must be born or at least a well-developed fetus to be a human being, then we might expect to see God only appearing in a late stage of development. It is hard to imagine God taking on some form that could have been discarded, ethically, as a mere blob of material.

In the first chapter of Luke we see Mary becoming pregnant with Jesus through the miraculous act of God. "Immediately," according to the text, she makes what was probably a several-day journey to visit her relative Elizabeth. Elizabeth's baby leaps in her womb at the encounter with Jesus as an embryo only a few days old and with the woman carrying him in her womb. In fact, Elizabeth addresses Mary as Jesus' mother. So Scripture emphasizes that not only is Jesus' presence already a reality, Mary's role and responsibility as his mother is as well.

This picture of responsibility for a human being even in one's weakest and most vulnerable states fits perfectly with the overall thrust of Scripture. We repeatedly find variations of the Proverbs 31:8-9 mandate to "speak up for those who cannot speak for themselves. . . . defend the rights of the poor and needy."

As we saw in chapter 3, our greatest bioethical challenge, second only to loving God, is to love our neighbor. That neighbor, as Jesus illustrates through the Good Samaritan story in Luke 10, is not merely someone who is like us. Rather, it is one who seems very different from us—one who is weak and vulnerable and utterly dependent on us if she or he is to live—one who our culture tells us can even be experienced at times as an enemy. (The man beaten helpless was a Jew but the helper was a Samaritan, and the two did not typically hold much good will toward one another.)

What an apt description of the embryo in our day! But rather than the embryo's utter dependence and lack of capability suggesting that we therefore have less responsibility, it suggests precisely that we have more. The very God of the universe became an embryo—a state we, too, have all gone through. If we are glad that we were not left unprotected, if we are glad that we were not seen as non-human beings, unworthy of protection, then what would it mean to love our neighbor as ourselves? What would it look like if we did to the embryo as we would have wanted done to us?

Concrete Bioethical Implications

Science and Scripture make compelling cases that embryos (and therefore fetuses as well) are human beings and worthy of the same treatment we give other human beings. However, we live in a world in which many do not recognize this to be true. In abortion-related cases since *Roe v. Wade,* the U.S. Supreme Court has been a voice for such people by affirming that we must proceed on the basis of uncertainty regarding whether or not embryos and fetuses are human beings.

What are the implications of such uncertainty? To answer this question we need only consider other situations in life in which there is uncertainty about whether or not a human being is present. How do we behave in such situations?

For example, if there is a forest in back of our house and we know that a child is not likely to be playing there at night—but could be, hidden from our view—we will not fire a gun into the trees. We do not reason that since it is not clear that a child is there, it is OK to fire. The possibility that a human being may be present is enough to restrain us. So if scientific or scriptural considerations even raise a question about whether or not a human being is present from fertilization onward, then honesty compels us to be cautious. We must not do anything that would endanger the life of an embryo unless we would do the same to any other human being. We should also do all we can to *support* the lives of embryos as well as other human beings.

In the arena of stem cell research, that means we should enthusiastically applaud adult stem cell research, but we should energetically oppose embryonic stem cell research. Adult stem cell research will probably greatly benefit ill people in the future without harming anyone in the process. In biblical terms it is "doing good" as we are commended to do (Galatians 6:10). However, embryonic stem cell research will necessarily destroy embryonic human beings in its attempt to help others. Biblically, it is "doing evil that good may result" as we are warned not to do (Romans 3:8).

As suggested earlier, fetal stem cell research may ethically resemble either adult or embryonic stem cell research and must be evaluated accordingly. If fetal stem cells are obtained from miscarried or stillborn fetuses, or if it becomes possible to remove them from fetuses still alive in the womb without harming the fetuses, then no harm is done to the donor and such fetal stem cell research can be wonderful. However, if the abortion of fetuses is the means by which fetal stem cells are obtained, then an unethical means (the killing of human beings) is involved. As explained in chapter 2, once we start thinking that "the ends justify the means," then we are subject to all the difficulties and dangers of an approach to bioethics that mistakenly thinks that good consequences are enough to justify anything.

In the arena of abortion, the implications are similar. We should enthusiastically do all we can

to support women who are pregnant under difficult circumstances. Meanwhile, we should energetically oppose killing their innocent unborn
children as a means of providing such support.
(The only embryos and fetuses who could be considered non-innocent are those who will cause
the death of their mother unless they are removed
from the mother's body. In that case, many people would say that removal, without killing if
possible, would be warranted, in defense of the
innocent life of the mother. Total pacifists, who
oppose all fighting even when one is being unjustly attacked, would not allow this exception.
Needless to say, the development of the artificial
womb will have great bearing on this matter.)

It is essential, in our approach to these and
other bioethical issues, that we are as clear about
what we are "for" as what we are "against." We
do need to know the cliffs to avoid, as explained
in chapter 3, so that in our love for people we can
steer them away from injuring themselves or
those who are with them. Even then, we should
not merely be "against" destroying embryos. We
should also be "for" efforts to enable infertile couples longing for children to adopt and give birth
to "unwanted" embryos left over from assisted re-

production attempts. The possibility of embryo adoption is a wonderful prospect that has only recently become an option (see chapter 7). Once we have avoided the cliffs, we are then left with the primary work of bioethics and of life. We must love our neighbors, as God enables and directs in the midst of challenges to life and health.

In particular, we must care for those who pay the price when tough ethical decisions are made. There is a woman in need if she decides not to abort her unwanted child. There is a man with Alzheimer's disease in need if he rejects a treatment that was developed from embryonic stem cell research—or if society decides not to pursue such research in the first place.

Human dignity, rooted in God's creation and incarnation, demands that we take the initiative in all situations such as these to identify the specific financial, emotional, spiritual, and other supports that suffering people and those around them need. Bearing one another's burdens in this way is more than calling attention to bioethical standards—it is making it possible to live by them.

5 Life on the Line: End-of-Life Treatment and Resource Allocation

Both of this book's authors have experienced loved ones going through the process of dying. For a while, certain treatments provided a hope of cure. Eventually, it became clear that our loved ones would die soon regardless of what was done.

One vivid situation involved one of our fathers who had been on and off the ventilator to enable him to breathe. Of all the treatments he had endured, he hated the ventilator more than anything. It helped his breathing by forcing air into his lungs, but it prevented him from speaking and was very uncomfortable. Now, as his death approached, his lungs began to fill with fluid for what would likely be the last time. Should the family put him back on the ventilator? Should we give him aggressive pain medication if there was a chance that doing so would relax his breathing so much that death might occur sooner as a result? Should we attempt one more hugely expensive experimental treatment that had little chance of working? Could we safely assume that he

would want us to bear this decision-making burden for him?

These are really tough decisions, and they are
as unavoidable as death itself. Today there are
wonderful life-sustaining technologies such as
ventilators to breathe for us, and dialysis machines to do the blood-cleansing work of our kid-
neys for us. But we have learned that these
machines, like any human invention, can be used
to help or harm us. Depending on our medical
condition, they can enable us to live, or they can
make an inescapable dying process even more
burdensome and painful.

So we need some basis for deciding how to care
for people appropriately when their health seriously deteriorates, particularly when death may
be approaching. What does a biblical perspective
offer us that other ways of looking at life do not?

As we saw in chapter 2, many people approach
life with a focus on consequences. In a potentially
end-of-life situation, they instinctively look at
the well-being of everyone affected, to see how
the greatest amount of well-being overall can be
preserved or produced. Whatever will lessen the
burden on the patient—all else being equal—
they see as good. This outlook may lead to aggres-

sive palliative care (relief of pain and suffering). However, it may also lead to letting the person die much earlier than necessary. If the burden on others or on the resources of the health care system will be eased by the person's death, then so much greater the reason for the premature death. As explained earlier, this is both a dangerous and impractical way to approach ethical decisions.

We also saw in chapter 2 that many today are influenced by an autonomy-based outlook. Such people make end-of-life judgments and all other decisions based on whatever they personally judge to be right. Such an approach is inadequate since it typically provides people with no *basis* for deciding, for example, when life-sustaining treatment should be withheld or stopped. It is preoccupied with procedural issues such as who should make the decisions and under what conditions they should make them. In fact, it really is dangerous because it allows fallen, self-centered people to define as right anything that suits their interests. It points people away from God by denying the validity of the God-established truths about people and life that must guide our actions if we are truly to flourish.

In line with our discussion in chapter 3, a biblical approach to end-of-life care avoids the pit-falls of other approaches by urging us to consider several matters when a person's death is in view. Those who love God will first want to glorify him by ensuring that any action they take or omit is in harmony with how God has created and intended the world to be. Concretely, because life is a pre-cious gift of God, nothing should be either done or omitted with the intention of promoting death. Also, because people have a God-given responsi-bility for their lives, no treatment or other inter-vention should be forced on people against their wishes if they are mentally competent. If an ac-tion we are considering involves intending death or violating the patient's wishes in this way, then it is wrong.

However, if more than one option before us does not involve either of these problems—or anything else immoral—then those who love their neighbors will pursue the option that will contribute most to human well-being, especially the patient's. A fuller discussion of the require-ments of love and human well-being will be re-served for the next chapter. The remainder of this chapter will explain the first two ethical require-ments for end-of-life decision making. It will then conclude with a look at how financial considerations complicate the picture.

Is Death Intended?

The most striking feature of end-of-life decisions is that, quite literally, life is on the line. What we decide to do—or not do—may result in the patient's death. So it is essential to have a clear understanding of what death is and what our attitude should be toward it. (We are addressing here the death of "innocent" people—patients—and not criminals or soldiers.)

Some today would say that death is simply a natural part of life, to be pursued at the appropriate time. Others would say that it is an ultimate evil, to be resisted at all costs. The first view can lead to undertreatment (or suicide), when people assume the responsibility to decide when they should die. The second view can lead to overtreatment, when a patient remains burdened by various tubes and technologies "to the bitter end," even though it is evident that life cannot be extended.

The biblical view is different from both of these popular perspectives. In the opening chapters of Genesis we find that death (understood both as physical and spiritual) entered the world because of people's disobedience and selfishness (2:17; 3:19). When people disobeyed God and went their own way, they were separated from God's life-giving power (the tree of life) which otherwise would have sustained them forever (3:22). Death, then, is an enemy—something contrary to that which God originally intended.

When we turn to the New Testament, we still find death portrayed as an enemy: "the last enemy to be destroyed" after Christ returns (1 Corinthians 15:26). It remains an enemy because it is the opposite of life and is a source of great sorrow and separation. As an enemy it is not something for us to support or encourage. Nevertheless, death is a *defeated enemy*. The resurrection of Jesus Christ from the dead has already demonstrated that eternal life triumphs over physical death, and that we need not desperately resist death as if we were facing annihilation.

What are the practical implications of seeing death as a defeated enemy—not to be intended but also not to be frantically opposed? First, if we are not to align ourselves with death by intending it, then we must first be clear, in any situation of illness or injury, whether continued living is an option. In some situations there will be a significant likelihood that patients can continue to live for years as long as they receive all available treatments. To withhold or withdraw life-sustaining treatment would unacceptably involve intending death. If it is impossible to gauge whether or not patients will continue to live with treatment, then withholding or withdrawing life-sustaining treatment would be similarly problematic.

> The resurrection of Jesus Christ from the dead has already demonstrated that eternal life triumphs over physical death, and that we need not desperately resist death as if we were facing annihilation.

However, in some situations, those with medical expertise have enough information and experience to recognize that a particular patient is in a "dying process." That means there is definitive evidence that the patient will die soon regardless of what treatments are continued (for example, if major organ systems are shutting down). When such is the case, then particular medical technologies such as the ventilator or dialysis machine may be withheld or withdrawn if they are adding more burden than benefit to the dying process.

Life cannot continue significantly longer regardless of treatment, so there need be no intention of death motivating the forgoing of treatment. If continued life is not a possibility, then patients should receive only treatment that supports rather than burdens them in the dying process.

While being in a dying process is not a neat and precise category, it is important that it not be too vague. People who may well live for years longer with treatment are not in a dying process as that term is used here. To deny them life-sustaining treatment would be to intend their death, since continued living is a possibility for them. Instead, only those patients who are imminently dying are in view here. Hospice programs, where life-sustaining treatments are discontinued and palliative care is central, are only for those in a dying process. How long a person will live under such conditions is rarely clear. But if there is reason to think that a patient's final dying days could well extend beyond a few weeks or months, then that patient is generally not admitted.

Psychologically it may be easier to withhold treatment in the first place than to withdraw it after it has begun. However, withholding is no more ethical than withdrawing. If anything, it may be less ethical, since it is not always clear in advance whether or not a possible treatment will actually help the patient. Trying a treatment and deciding later not to continue it if it definitely proves ineffective is more justifiable than not starting it just because it might be ineffective. Far more lives will be lost with the second approach than with the first.

Sadly, the development of wonderful technologies has partly shifted people's focus from the patient to the patient-attached-to-technology. It seems at times that it is as hard to disconnect machines from patients as it would be to cut off their arms or legs. That should not be. Our focus must be squarely on patients. If their well-being is not best served by a technology, then they must be spared from it, whether they are already connected to it or not. Knowing that withdrawing a treatment is psychologically difficult, we would do well to insist on a trial period for a technology when its benefit is uncertain—much like we take prescription medicine for a disease. Just as we do not renew the prescription unless more medicine is needed, so we can decide in advance not to continue the technology beyond the trial period unless benefit is likely.

Some may wonder about the morality of giving pain medication aggressively if it might relax the patient enough that death occurs a little sooner. Again, the question "Is death intended?" can be our guide. If the dose given is higher than the minimum necessary to relieve the pain, then the fatal intention is evident and the action is immoral. But if the honest intention is pain relief and not death, then necessary medication is justified. In fact, while it is conceivable that the resulting relaxation could lead to a slightly earlier death, it is far more likely that relief from the ravages of pain will enable the body to live longer.

Is the Patient Willing?

Even informed by the same counsel, people may reach different decisions (see chapter 2). So another unavoidable issue in medical treatment is who should make the decision. From a biblical perspective the decision to treat or not to treat rests ultimately with the patient.

In end-of-life treatment, it is especially apparent that life is on the line—the patient's life. So the question then becomes: Who is responsible for that life, and for the decisions that most profoundly affect it? The biblical mandate to "choose life" (see Deuteronomy 30:19) is especially relevant here, for the "life" in view, biblically, encompasses our physical as well as broader spiritual well-being. The mandate speaks not only to what we should

From a biblical perspective the decision to treat or not to treat rests ultimately with the patient.

choose, as already discussed, but also to who is responsible for the decision. When people's lives are at stake, people themselves must decide to pursue what they need in order to live. God will not force it on them against their will.

The eternal context of our lives sets the pattern for vital medical decisions. People have a God-given responsibility to make the right choice (that is, to follow Christ) if they are to live eternally with God. Similarly, the (ultimately less significant) responsibility to make decisions about medical treatment, whether life-sustaining or not, rests with those who must bear the consequences. We cannot force people to make wise choices—in matters of faith or in matters of physical well-being.

Nevertheless, those associated with patients do have a responsibility to help them make good decisions. That includes family members, friends, and, in the medical context, physicians

and others. In fact, to not question patients' expressed wishes to forgo treatment can easily
miscommunicate. If treatment can enable them to
continue living, our silence may confirm their
worst fears: that others don't consider their life
worth living. Health-related professionals have
the added obligation to make sure that patients
are truly capable of making decisions, as will be
discussed shortly.

Nevertheless, patients have primary (human)
responsibility for those decisions. That's why the
apostle Paul, in the midst of an extended plea for
people to "carry each other's burdens" (Galatians
6:2-10), rather unexpectedly insists that "each
one should carry his own load" (v. 5). Each person has the ultimate human responsibility for the
life God gives her or him, and others should provide the support needed to fulfill that responsibility, not take that responsibility away.

That we are responsible does not mean that our
decisions are always right. Today's popular autonomy ethics says that whatever I decide is right
for me, *is* right, simply because I judge it to be so.
The biblical outlook says that the basis of right
and wrong is outside of ourselves—that we are
morally accountable to standards beyond our-

selves. Accordingly, it is possible for us to make wrong decisions. But they are ours to make. So whether we choose or refuse what will give us eternal life or life in this world (that is, medical treatment), the decision is ours and is not to be made for us—even if we decide wrongly. Since we may make wrong decisions, however, others have the obligation to try to persuade us to decide rightly.

Practically speaking, how do we know patients' wishes? If possible, we ask them. But there are four important ethical safeguards to insure that what patients say reflects their true wishes. First, they must have the mental capacity to make a decision. This means that they are able to take in information, assess it in relation to their beliefs and values, and communicate the resulting decision. Not only unconsciousness, but also other conditions such as depression can undermine people's decision-making capacity. It is a caregiver's—especially a physician's—responsibility to be sure that a patient is mentally capable, and that if capability is limited, everything possible is done to restore that capability before important decisions are made.

Second, patients must be free from coercion.

That includes not only the coercion of family members or health care professionals, but also the coercive force of such factors as money. Sometimes monetary considerations limit treatment options, but that constraint should not be confused with what the patient genuinely wants apart from such considerations. Third, patients must receive the information they need in order to make a good decision. They need information about their condition, their likely future without treatment, and their likely futures with each possible treatment (including possible harms and benefits).

Yet, all too often, patients are given an inadequate "informed consent" document to sign, containing only information regarding the treatment option being recommended. Furthermore, even that information may be in hard-to-read small print using words that are difficult to understand. That's why a fourth ethical safeguard requires that patients have not only information but also understanding. If there are statistical risks of danger, for example, people need to understand how those compare to risks they are more familiar with in everyday life.

Otherwise, they may have the experience one

of the present authors had when his wife developed a health problem. She was advised to have a treatment, one whose possible outcome was simply listed as "death." As soon as that word was read, the decision-making process screeched to a halt inside of them. Had they been told that there was roughly the same likelihood of death as being hit by a car on their next cross-country driving trip, they could have understood the risk and not been overwhelmed by it.

A relatively simple way for a caregiver or friend to determine if patients' decisions meet these four ethical criteria is to ask them what they have decided and why. If they cannot give any explanation that reflects their personal values, then they may lack decision-making capacity, may have been subtly coerced, or, most likely, were given information but not helped to understand that information well enough to reach a genuinely informed decision. When information or understanding is lacking, it must be adequately provided so that the patient can make an ethical decision concerning treatment.

However, what happens when patients have lost decision-making ability and it cannot be restored? In that case, patients are best served if they have a certain type of "advance directive" through which their wishes can still be respected.

When information or understanding is lacking, it must be adequately provided so that the patient can make an ethical decision concerning treatment.

One popular form of advance directive is the "living will" in which people write down various types of treatments they do or don't want under circumstances that they specify. However, such documents by themselves are risky, because it is impossible to know the future. Living wills may include a sweeping statement about a technology the patient *never* wants, yet some unusual temporary need for that technology may arise that the patient would have approved.

For that reason, a better type of advance directive has emerged, the "durable power of attorney for health care." It enables people simply to specify who they want to make treatment decisions for them (their "surrogate decision-maker") if they lose the capacity to do so. That way, someone who understands their wishes can make needed decisions in specific situations.

People are welcome to include in their advance directive some written advice to their surrogate, as long as it is clear that it is advice only and that the surrogate's judgment takes priority. Otherwise, the living will directions in the advance directive may come into direct conflict with what the surrogate knows the patient would have wanted, and these directions may hinder carrying out the decision the patient truly would have wanted. It is also important that written advice not take the place of lengthier and more nuanced discussions between patients and their surrogates (and possibly backup surrogates as well).

What happens when a patient has lost decision-making capacity but has no advance directive? Ethically, the standard is still to follow the patient's wishes. If those can't be determined, then the standard becomes the "best interests" of the patient, as best those can be identified. Accordingly, many states specify a hierarchy of surrogate decision makers such as spouses and other close relations, ranked on the basis of how in touch they typically are with patients' wishes or interests.

To summarize, then: to be ethical, end-of-life treatment decisions must not intend death or force treatment on patients against their wishes. As noted previously, however, there is much more to ethical end-of-life care than this. Since good end-of-life care, though, is the primary alternative to assisted suicide, it is better to postpone further discussion until the next chapter.

Does the Cost Matter?

To this point, we have been talking as if the cost of treatment does not matter. If something might benefit the patient and the patient wants it, then the patient gets it. If only it were that simple!

Few people have medical blank checks at their disposal, unless they are wealthy. The reason for this bad news is the good news that so much is available in health care today. But some of it is very expensive. Health care at the end of life is particularly expensive, because of the monitoring, the life support equipment, and the increasingly radical interventions that must be tried as the patient's condition grows worse.

So we recognize today that everyone can't receive every possible high-cost, high-tech intervention, particularly when there is only an extremely small chance that there will be a very small benefit from it. Every country in the world could be spending an enormous portion of its resources on health care, to the detriment of everything else. There are, after all, other needs in life besides health care.

At the same time, one might well argue that far greater health care expenditures than we make today are warranted. For example, a recent study has noted a striking result of placing such tight financial limits on one crucial resource, hospital personnel: There are an estimated 75,000 preventable deaths each year in the U.S. alone due to infections that patients acquire *from* hospitals. Furthermore, a relatively modest investment of resources could prevent far greater numbers of people from dying of measles, malaria, or lack of prenatal care in less developed countries all over the world. Nevertheless, until we allocate much more to health care, we have to decide how best to spend the available resources.

Aware of resource limitations, people will look at a dying man who needs a hugely expensive intervention and ask, *Is he worth it?* Or they will look at conjoined twin girl infants who must be separated at the cost of a million dollars if both are to live, and ask, *Are they worth it?* To answer this question, we must be very careful to distinguish three issues that often get confused: the benefit issue, the risk issue, and the allocation issue.

The *benefit issue* is the matter of whether or not patients' lives can be extended or their health improved with treatment. How much is a life worth? A thousand dollars? A million dollars? Biblically, as we saw in chapter 3, life is not something we put on a monetary scale along with the satisfaction of eating an ice cream cone and every other good consequence we can produce with our money. The mandate to support human life goes beyond monetary trade-offs of this kind. We should answer, without hesitation, that of course the man's life and the twins' lives are each worth a million dollars—and more. To hesitate in giving this answer is to reveal an unbiblical outlook on the great significance of human beings created in God's image.

Aware of resource limitations, people will look at a dying man who needs a hugely expensive intervention and ask, *Is he worth it?*

However, the second issue—*the risk issue*—requires us to say more. Treatment may involve possible benefits to life and health, but serious burdens may be involved as well. A treatment that could enable us to live for several years longer might add nothing to our life span but instead cause our dying to be more uncomfortable. We have no obligation to pursue treatment that will make our lives worse rather than better.

So we have to assess how great and how likely are the possible benefits and possible harms of treatment. Then we have to decide how much of a risk we are willing to take. How much harm are we willing to risk in order for benefit to be possible? Because the patient will be the primary one to experience any harms that result, the patient must be the one to decide whether or not the risk is worth taking. If the treatment in view can be life-sustaining and the possible harms are minimal, then there is little risk and we have an ethical mandate to "choose life." But where the risk is significant, this mandate does not settle the issue, and the patient's judgment, in consultation with others, is key.

Allocation Priorities

Even when a treatment may well be beneficial and taking the risk is justified, there remains another matter: *the allocation issue*. Because so many potential uses for our health care dollars are worthwhile, we must have ways to prioritize. But who should do this prioritizing?

Patients, first of all, are in no position to prioritize all of society's resources when they are ill. They can make their own resources available to pay for needed health care, to the extent that meeting other vital needs is not jeopardized as a result. But to whatever extent they need their insurance company or the hospital or the government to cover the cost, they simply do not have enough information to determine how their personal health care needs compare to the needs of everyone else. Nor does the physician, nor do other members of the health care team. All that the patient and health care team can be expected to do is to try to obtain any health care that will likely be beneficial and not too risky for the patient. If a treatment meets those criteria, patients and their caregivers should not feel bad in the least about doing all they can (ethically) to obtain it.

The responsibility for setting allocation priorities lies elsewhere, depending on their type. Priorities can be *macro* (big) or *micro* (small). (Sometimes the term *meso* [middle] is used for priorities that are set within specific government or private health care institutions such as the National Institutes of Health or a local hospital.)

Macro priorities govern many decisions at the international, national, state/regional, and local levels. A government, health care institution, or funding/insurance organization typically makes such decisions.

Macro decisions can involve determining how much of the total resources should go toward promoting life and health, as opposed to other worthy goals. They can involve judging how much of the health-related resources should be devoted directly to health care as opposed to other activities that directly affect health—for example, protecting the environment and promoting healthy lifestyles. They can involve allocating the resulting health care resources among competing priorities such as disease prevention, treatment of illness, and long-term care. And even within one of these priorities—to take treatment of illness as an example—they can involve allocating resources among all of the possible treatments.

The ethical challenge here is to find an appropriate way to make these various macro allocations. One of the first ways developed has been dubbed "cost-benefit analysis." In this approach, every benefit and cost is converted into the same unit—often dollars. That way, a single total number (benefits minus costs) can be attached to each possible treatment. For example, if prenatal care provided by a clinic will cost $1.4 million but will generate $2.6 million worth of benefit in reduced premature infant health care and less stress and health risk to mothers, then the high positive number of 1.2 (2.6 minus 1.4) million will be assigned to prenatal care. The higher the treatment's total number, the higher an allocation priority it receives. People have found, however, that it is impossible to convert all costs and benefits (especially benefits) accurately into dollars. Many have also observed that the method provides no way to ensure the benefits are distributed fairly among people.

So another approach has surpassed it in popularity, so-called "cost-effectiveness analysis." In this approach, benefits do not have to be measured in dollars. Rather, a more appropriate single standard just for benefits can be used. Since medical benefit is a matter of longer life and better health, some have suggested a standard that assigns a score to each treatment reflecting its impact on quality as well as length of life.

This approach, too, has its limitations—and not just the difficulty of finding an exact formula for generating these scores accurately. The problem of how to ensure a fair distribution of benefits remains. There is also the added difficulty that it is biased against treatments for the illnesses of older people, who will not normally live as long following treatment as others. (For that reason, the scores given to their treatments will necessarily be lower.) This is no small matter, in light of God's concern for older people: "Even to your old age and gray hairs I am he, I am he who will sustain you" (Isaiah 46:4), and "Rise in the presence of the aged, show respect for the elderly and revere your God. I am the Lord" (Leviticus 19:32). Such biblical affirmation contrasts sharply with the disregard that Israel's enemies have for older people (see Deuteronomy 28:50; 2 Chronicles 36:17; Lamentations 5:12).

In the end, there may be no single approach that directly produces ideal macro allocations. Rather, some approach such as cost-effectiveness analysis needs to be used, with the most accurate formula we can devise. The results then need to be adjusted, as necessary, to compensate for unjust outcomes.

Macro priorities are not the only challenge here. After they are in place, and we know how many resources will be available for particular treatments in particular institutions or regions, micro priorities are also necessary. These govern decisions about which particular patients will receive any treatment that is limited. Such micro allocations are necessary not only when macro allocations have provided insufficient resources to treat everyone in need. They are also necessary when a resource is naturally or temporarily scarce.

For example, thousands of people in the U.S. alone die annually because not enough organs such as hearts and livers are donated for transplantation. And just as there were many years before the expensive new artificial kidney (dialysis machine) could be made available to all who needed it in order to live, so will likely be the scenario if the totally implantable artificial heart is perfected. Who should live when not all can live? Who are the two people sitting closest to you at the moment? If you could save the life of only one, whom would you choose? How would you decide? (You would refuse to decide? Then you would let both die? Probably not.)

Those today guided by the popular but dangerous ethics of consequences (see chapter 2) would say that those most valuable to society should have top priority. When the artificial kidney was first developed, whether patients lived or died often depended on how beneficial to society a hospital's selection committee judged them to be. Discriminatory considerations such as race and age had great influence.

An approach with such biblical concerns as freedom, life, and justice, as well as broader social benefit (see chapter 3), advocates a different set of priorities. Biblical justice in particular essentially requires that those who want a scarce treatment that is essential to sustain their lives should be given an equal opportunity to receive it (even by some form of random selection, if necessary). Those who know God recognize the high priority God places on justice (Psalm 99:4; Jeremiah 9:24; 22:15-16). Jesus singles it out as a particularly important ethical concern (Matthew 23:23; Luke 11:42). Paul notes that the equal importance of the lives of everyone means that there must be equal access where life-sustaining resources are at stake (2 Corinthians 8:13-14).

The only exception in today's health care allocation would be if giving special priority to some would ultimately result in more lives overall being saved. Such is rarely the case, but allocating one available dialysis machine to many who need it only temporarily rather than to one who needs it permanently would be an example. The more essential a treatment is for sustaining life itself, the more applicable the call of justice to meet people's life-threatening needs equally.

Detailing the general macro and micro priorities introduced here is not something that patients or caregivers should attempt to do once the patients have become ill and need treatment. It is a vital activity that must be done in advance by society, communities, and institutions. Nevertheless, health care professionals, particularly physicians, know more about the medical issues involved in such priority setting than virtually anyone else. So while it remains true that physicians should not attempt to judge whether or not a patient's life is "worth" the cost of a possible but expensive treatment, more must be said. It is equally true that physicians should be among the most active participants in determining general macro and micro priorities.

Patients, meanwhile, can participate in broader priority setting as well. But they, too, should not undermine respect for human life generally—not to mention respect for their own lives—by attempting to judge if their lives are worth the cost of treatment. Rather, they should be assessing the benefits of treatment, and the risks of resulting harms outweighing the benefits. They must make the initial decision for or against treatment—a decision that biblically should intend life rather than death. However, at that point their treatment becomes subject to any allocation priorities that limit what their health care team can do for them.

If limited resources have been allocated to their form of treatment, then they might die. However, it is important for everyone to be clear that allocation priorities are responsible for this tragedy. Patients, physicians, and others are sometimes tempted to let society off the hook by making judgments about whether saving a patient's life is "worth it" (to refer back to our earlier examples of the dying man and the conjoined twins). If people are willing to do that, then there is no reason for society to do anything more in support of human life and health. Only those who are "worth it" are being treated.

However, people must refuse to do that. They must require society to provide life-sustaining resources to patients who will die without them. That changes the picture entirely. Society will have to make sure that its allocations are generous enough to give adequate respect to human life and health. Certain scarcities will disappear with the increased funding that will result, as will the tragic micro allocations they require.

6 Breathtaking Decisions: Assisted Suicide and Euthanasia

We opened the previous chapter with the experience one of our families had making difficult end-of-life treatment decisions with a parent. There was more to that story. As all involved looked to the final suffering that lay ahead, visions of the worst situations we had seen on television or heard about in the news or from friends filled our minds. If death was inevitable fairly soon, and suffering was likely, then might it not be the most compassionate option to ask the physician to give Dad some medicine that would end his life right away? One or two family members in particular expressed how hard it was to watch Dad deteriorate. Why not spare everyone the suffering that lay ahead?

At the patient's bed that day, where any decision would have to be implemented, three parties had a particular stake in the decision-making process. There was the physician, who represented what health care with its team of professionals could contribute to the situation. There were the patient and his loved ones, who were suffering. And there was the heavenly Father, who loved the patient, family, and physician with a love surpassing all human love. In order to answer the questions tugging at the hearts and minds of those involved in the tough decision making involved here, it is important to consider the situation from the perspective of each of these parties. We will look first at assisted suicide, where the patient is the one who causes the death (for example, by taking a fatal medication). Then we will consider euthanasia, where a person other than the patient directly causes the patient's death.

What's at Stake for Health Care?

What does the option of physician-assisted suicide look like, first of all, from the physician's perspective? What is at stake for health care as a whole, embodied here by the physician? Health care has long had two core commitments: sustaining life and relieving suffering. The idea that a person could relieve suffering by ending life is not new. If anything, that idea was more plausible in an earlier age before the wonderful pain management we have today became available.

Nevertheless, as discussed in chapter 1, health care has steadfastly held the two together—committed to relieving as much suffering as possible while working to sustain life if possible.

A serious problem with physician-assisted suicide is that it pursues one of these core commitments, relieving suffering, directly at the expense of the other core commitment, sustaining life. So it destroys the essential character and foundation of health care. It represents the end of health care as we have known it.

What does this mean, practically speaking? Perhaps you've seen the picture of the patient in the Oregon hospital who has just read a newspaper account of

A serious problem with physician-assisted suicide is that it pursues one of these core commitments, relieving suffering, directly at the expense of the other core commitment, sustaining life.

the legalization of physician-assisted suicide there. Instead of being reassured by a button at his bedside to call the health care team if needed, he is clutching the hot button to the police! Pictured here is the breakdown in trust that is unavoidable when patients can no longer count on health care as an institution that stands consistently for the sustaining of life. If assisted suicide is an option that health care provides, then health care sometimes is an agent of life and sometimes an agent of death.

Some will protest, of course, that patients can still rely on health care professionals to sustain their lives. The only instances in which the health care team would help cause patients' deaths, they insist, would be if numerous, carefully worded medical and other criteria are met. However, we need to be realistic here. When patients are sick and weak, they are in no condition to remember a list of criteria and to determine whether or not they fit the criteria—every hour! It doesn't matter how simple and personal the criteria are.

Even limiting assisted suicide to cases where the patient gives consent means that assisted suicide is sometimes possible. With the awareness of that reality comes the knowledge that there is some situation in which the patient's own physician can try to bring about the patient's death. Patients are far less likely to be able to remember what the specific criteria are—no matter what they are—than they are to know in a simple, straightforward way what health care stands for. Either it stands without question or exception for the sustaining of life, or it does not. If physician-assisted suicide is an option, it does not.

So health care professionals should be among the first in line to oppose the practice of physician-assisted suicide. The very integrity and trustworthiness of health care itself is at stake.

What's at Stake for Patients and Their Loved Ones?

Patients and their loved ones should be right near the front of the line with the professionals—for the same reasons, and more. At stake is far more than their ability to trust their physicians and health care teams, as important as that is. How effectively their own pressing needs are met is also on the line. In order to understand this, it will help to review what these needs are. When we see how ineffectively these needs are sometimes met today, we can better understand why so many people are open to the assisted-suicide option.

First of all, patients need adequate health care. However, in the United States alone, over 40 million people are without any health insurance to cover the cost of their health care. Wonderfully, many health care professionals and institutions provide substantial care without charge to those who cannot pay, and many patients have the financial ability to pay for their own health care. So studies have been done to determine if lack of health insurance for many actually means that a significant number of people get much sicker and even die as a result. The answer turns out to be yes. The first need that patients have, then, is for adequate health care—and a significant number today are not receiving it.

Next, once patients have adequate health care in general, it is essential that they have adequate pain management in particular. But studies continue to show that many do not. For example, one recent study found that about half of the half-million patients who die from cancer each year in the U.S. receive no pain and symptom management at all. Sometimes the reason is that their physicians' training (often decades ago) included little instruction in pain control. When that is the case, physicians may pay too little attention to relieving a patient's symptoms because they are so focused on curing or improving the patient's medical condition. In other cases, physicians may be reluctant to allow patients to have as much pain medication as the patients want, out of concern that they will become addicted or will lose their alertness.

A third pressing need that goes unmet for some is adequate suffering management. People may have effective pain control, but suffering is different from pain. Whereas pain is a physical sensation, suffering involves a threat to one's identity— one's sense of worth and meaning in life. It is possible to experience suffering without having any physical pain, just as it is possible to experience pain without suffering. What is needed in the face of suffering is not just pain medication, but counsel and support—emotional, spiritual, and otherwise. That is why health care teams are so important, in order to provide suffering patients and their loved ones with the support they need. Not only physicians, nurses, and physician assistants are needed, but also chaplains, social workers, and others.

This wholistic team approach, attending to the full range of human needs, has been the source of the hospice movement's success. Hospice care— either in the home or in a health care institution—focuses exclusively on helping patients to die well rather than continuing medical attempts to prevent death. It is a wonderful option for those who have entered the dying process described in chapter 5. But it is not an option always offered to patients who need it.

Finally, when patients are dying they need assurance that they are in control of the health care decisions that are having such an impact on their lives. They rightly consider these decisions to be their responsibility, as we saw in the previous chapter. But they know that there can be such a focus on curative medicine at the expense of symptom relief—and legal worries on the part of some health care professionals and institutions—that unwanted treatments can be started at any time. They also know that stopping treatment already begun can be next to impossible.

Patients need to know that their values and wishes will be respected in the dying process. That is important not only when they are still able to express them, but also after they lose their mental capacity. Advance directives (see chapter 5) arose to give people assurance in this area. But those

Patients need to know that their values and wishes will be respected in the dying process.

who have the living will form of directive instinctively know that living wills do not cover every possible scenario. So they are only partly reassuring. Moreover, studies continue to show that patients' wishes expressed in advance directives are not being consulted in a significant number of cases.

There are four major ways, then, in which patients need support near the end of their lives: adequate health care, adequate pain relief, adequate suffering management, and adequate attention to their wishes. In other words, people need support. The need is not for a new form of independence—for a life-ending autonomy—as proponents of assisted suicide would suggest. So much of contemporary Western culture is awash in autonomy (see chapter 2)—in an individualism that does not engage people in fulfilling the needs and wishes of others but separates people from one another. It desensitizes people to the need that others have for their care.

Assisted suicide responds to this predicament by fanning the flames of the fire. In effect, it encourages the current lack of support by cutting people off from any further need for support. It is the perfect quick fix in a fast food society. Get rid of the suffering by getting rid of the sufferer. It does a grave disservice to whatever efforts are underway to improve the supports desperately needed by suffering and dying patients. Providing such supports truly respects patients and enhances their freedom—the very goals autonomy claims to champion. If society can instead get rid of problems by getting rid of patients, then there is far less need to develop the ability to meet patients' real needs.

Why Does All This Matter to God?

To this point we have made several key observations about assisted suicide. Particularly when a physician provides the assistance, it is very much against the interests of physicians and other health care professionals, as well as contrary to the interests of patients and their loved ones. But what does such an act look like to our heavenly Father, who is as present at the patient's bedside as any physician or family member?

In the previous chapter we discussed two biblical criteria for good end-of-life decisions. First, we noted that death should not be the intended result of any of our actions or inaction. Assisted suicide necessarily violates this standard, since death is precisely the intended outcome. It is a form of "taking my life into my own hands"—the very thing Job refused to do no matter how great his suffering (Job 13:13-15). At the end of his life, Paul models for us a similar willingness to live or die in the face of suffering, as God deems best, regardless of one's personal preferences: "that my life will always honor Christ, whether I live or I die" (Philippians 1:20, NLT). As he had previously reminded others that "you are not your own" (1 Corinthians 6:19), so he now affirms the same for himself. In this he follows Jesus. In the Garden of Gethsemane, Jesus was honest with his heavenly Father about his fervent desire to escape end-of-life suffering, but ultimately he decides "Not my will, but yours be done" (Luke 22:42).

Perhaps less apparent, however, is how assisted suicide can violate the second biblical criterion, that is, that the patient's wishes be respected. Remember that even if a patient were genuinely to want assisted suicide, it would be wrong because death would be intended. Yet in so many cases where assisted suicide is carried out or considered, the patient's wishes are not truly respected. Typically, that means one of the four requirements of an ethical "informed consent" discussed in chapter 5 is violated.

The first requirement is that patients have the

mental ability to make and communicate decisions in line with their true values and wishes.
All too often, though, people considering suicide
are seriously depressed, and depression can easily lead us to make decisions that we later regret
(if we are still alive) once the depression is gone.
The second requirement, that the decision be voluntary, can also be easily violated. One example
is when a patient feels pressure from the family to
stop being an emotional and financial drain on
them. Such pressure may be actual, because the
family does indeed want to be free from this burden and either communicates such a desire or is
unable to hide it. Or such pressure may be imagined by the patient, but there is no overt effort by
the family to persuade the patient that the fear is
groundless because the patient never expresses it
in the first place.

Perhaps the most commonly violated requirement of informed consent in assisted-suicide
cases is the requirement of information. Patients
are to be given information concerning their
"treatment" alternatives, which in this case
would include the option of assisted suicide. For
each alternative, such information must include a
description of what patients might well experi-

ence if that option is elected. The assisted-suicide option will involve death, so patients considering this option should in theory be given information about what death will be like for them.

What would such information include? There are certainly various religious and nonreligious views about what death will entail. But in a country like the United States, where the majority of the people claim to be Christians, the traditional Christian view of what death will entail should at least be a part of the information conveyed. In other words, patients should be informed about what death will be like for those who follow Christ, and for those who do not, according to the Bible. Needless to say, providing such information about what death will entail is not standard practice in health care. Truly informed consent to assisted suicide is not often obtained. Nevertheless, it is important to note that a caregiver or friend who lovingly conveys such information to a person considering assisted suicide is well within the bounds of what is called for in an informed consent process.

In still other cases of assisted suicide, the fourth requirement of informed consent—understanding—is violated. It is one thing to be told that a possible treatment option is to receive good pain and suffering management. It is another thing entirely to experience it. As explained above, people are aware that so many never receive such effective management. It only makes sense that they will not give this option the weight it deserves—even according to their own value system—unless they have experienced it for themselves. Patients cannot give an informed consent to assisted suicide without experiencing all forms of pain and suffering management that could reasonably help them.

At this point, a few comments on the difference between assisted suicide and euthanasia are important. We focus here primarily on assisted suicide, since that is the focus of debate in so many countries today. And if assisting someone to kill themselves is wrong, then it almost goes without saying that allowing someone other than the patient to kill the patient (euthanasia) would be wrong. However, the world's experience to date with euthanasia is instructive regarding the most important "safeguard" related to the practice of assisted suicide: the standard of informed consent. So some explicit attention to euthanasia is helpful.

Many people are most familiar with euthanasia from the role it played in Nazi Germany. It first involved killing physically and mentally weak people, and then included eliminating racially "undesired" people such as Jews. The term comes from two Greek words meaning "good death." "Euthanasia" suggests that the death involved is a good thing in general. But in Nazi Germany euthanasia was practiced for the supposed good of others or society in general, not for the good of the people killed.

For decades the atrocities of Nazi Germany, among other factors, discouraged other countries from allowing euthanasia. In recent years, however, The Netherlands has taken the lead in allowing euthanasia (first by agreeing not to punish some physicians who practiced it, and more recently by legalizing it). To do so, the country has had to reject, with Nazi Germany, the God-given mandate not to intend the death of an innocent person. Yet it has sought to avoid the horrors of Nazi Germany by requiring that euthanasia be practiced only when the patient explicitly requests it. (A similar direction has more recently been taken by Belgium and Colombia.)

It is instructive to see what happens in practice

once the absolute, clear protection of innocent human life ends. After euthanasia had been allowed for a number of years, the Dutch government conducted a study of its practice. The results of the study are contained in the official report of the Dutch Committee to Investigate the Medical Practice Concerning Euthanasia, released late in 1991. Since the study involved professionals reporting how ethical or unethical their use of it was, probably more ethical lapses existed than were reported. Even so, the study documented nearly 6,000 cases annually where patients were killed without their consent!

Once killing consenting patients was allowed, physicians soon began to consider another possibility. Since mentally incompetent (or unconscious) patients could not give their consent, some Dutch physicians reasoned, others should be allowed to make life-ending decisions for them. Until this point, the best protection patients had was the requirement that they must explicitly request euthanasia before it could be performed on them.

Now, with this protection gone, professionals began to make judgments about which incompetent patients would probably want to be killed.

So it was not surprising that, when they encountered competent patients in medical conditions similar to those of incompetent patients whom they had killed, they began to kill some of these competent patients as well without obtaining their consent. Thus, the Dutch study found that in nearly a quarter of the 6,000 cases where patients were killed without their consent, the patients were still mentally competent!

The Dutch experience is a vivid illustration of what can easily—perhaps inevitably—happen when it becomes acceptable to intend a patient's death. The informed consent requirement is not sufficient, in the real world, to insure that the patient's consent will be obtained. Once intending death is considered OK, it is sometimes easier for those who do the killing to judge for themselves who should die.

Accordingly, Oregon's relatively recent legalization of assisted suicide, as long as the patient consents, should concern us

> **O**nce intending death is considered OK, it is sometimes easier for those who do the killing to judge for themselves who should die.

greatly. Although the U.S. Supreme Court has rejected the idea that everyone has a "right to die" or a "right to assisted suicide"—and states are not rushing to follow Oregon's lead in legalizing assisted suicide—problems with the informed consent standard in Oregon have already begun to appear. One widely publicized case involved a situation in which the patient may well have been pressured into assisted suicide by a family member. Oregon physicians seldom call for psychiatric evaluations of patients who request assisted suicide, despite the fact that studies repeatedly have shown that physicians not trained in psychiatry are often unable to diagnose depression accurately. It is no wonder that a recent ABC News poll found support for assisted suicide in the U.S. lowest among older Americans. They are the ones who are most at risk if their lives are subject to the judgments of others concerning their mental ability or medical condition.

Those who are at the bedside with true compassion—as God is—will not enter into such judgments. They will heed God's mandate to "choose life" rather than intend death. But it is all too easy to conclude that a biblical perspective on assisted suicide and euthanasia is simply the warning that both are wrong. The problem with this view is that it limits people without pointing them to better alternatives. Such an approach is in flat contradiction to the Bible, where we learn that God expects us not only to live morally, but also to provide for one another the support and resources we need in order to so live.

There are very few things in the New Testament that have the force of law—that impose absolute requirements on our daily living. However, providing people what they need to remain true to God is one of them. As Paul expresses it, "Carry each other's burdens, and in this way you will fulfill the law of Christ" (Galatians 6:2). The *law* of Christ? Yes, the law— that which is essential, if people are to be able to honor God by making the best choices in tough situations. One such choice can be to reject assisted suicide and euthanasia.

If we are to make that choice, we will require the support of others. Some must provide or help us obtain essential health care including effective pain control. Others will need to insure that we participate appropriately in decision making. Still others will have to help us deal with the emotional and spiritual suffering that makes continuing to live so difficult.

All of this is what true compassion is about.

The word "compassion" comes from two Latin words meaning "suffering with"—which is precisely what we *stop* doing when we encourage or participate in assisted suicide or euthanasia. Biblical compassion is loving our neighbor concretely in a way that honors God. It always gives first priority to how God has created the world to be, urging that people take responsibility for their decisions and choose life. But then it actively goes to work doing all it can to meet the needs of people, who are, after all, created in God's own image (see chapter 3). Such compassion is what good end-of-life care requires, whether or not assisted suicide and euthanasia present a serious temptation.

PART THREE

□ □ □ □ □

BIOTECHNOLOGY:
Shaping the Human Race

7 Thirty-eight Ways to Make a Baby

There are as many as 6.1 million infertile couples in America—that's nearly the size of New York City. At the same time, there are at least thirty-eight ways to make a baby, if you consider all the possible configurations and therapies. Infertile couples are confronted with an alphabet soup of options including AIH, AID, GIFT, ZIFT, IVF, surrogacy, and others. With so many couples desiring children, and with so many options, making decisions about reproductive technologies can be extraordinarily difficult.

Low-tech Pregnancy

It is important at the outset to understand exactly what constitutes infertility. The diagnosis of infertility is made when a couple fails to achieve pregnancy after twelve months of unprotected sexual intercourse. Even under the best of circumstances there is only a 15 percent to 20 percent likelihood of pregnancy for "normal" couples having sex regularly.[1] In young women, the chance for pregnancy with unprotected intercourse is estimated at 20 percent each month, while for women over the age of forty, the chances are probably less than 5 percent each month.[2]

There are many things couples can do to improve their chances of getting pregnant. Couples should become familiar with their own reproductive cycles so as to take advantage of peak periods of fertility. Remember that the female's egg only lives for about twenty-four hours after it is released from her ovary.

Monitoring ovulation by keeping a basal body temperature chart can be very effective for some couples. Basal body temperature is body temperature when one first wakes up in the morning. Reading basal body temperature accurately requires a special thermometer available from a drug store. Even better is the use of over-the-counter ovulation predictor kits. The use of alcohol, tobacco, and high levels of stress can negatively impact one's ability to get pregnant. Couples who want to get pregnant and are having difficulty should consult their gynecologist or family physician for advice on how to get pregnant.

Husbands should realize that infertility is not merely the wife's "problem." In fact, in up to 30 percent of the cases of infertility so-called "male factors" are to blame. In another 30 percent of the cases a female factor makes pregnancy difficult to achieve. The remaining 40 percent of the cases of infertility are due to a combination of factors or to undetermined causes.[3]

High-tech Pregnancy

Reproductive technologies have come a very long way in a very short period of time. Since the 1970s the fertility industry has experienced explosive growth. The high-tech options for getting pregnant continue to expand.

Fertility drugs

The most common treatment for infertility is drug therapy. Problems with ovulation constitute the main reasons for infertility among women. Drugs such as Perganol may be used to cause "super-ovulation." That is, these drugs cause women to release more eggs than they would during a normal cycle.

Fertility drugs are normally safe, but may have side effects. One side effect is an increased likelihood of multiple births during the same pregnancy. The chances for multiple births increase about 25 percent when super-ovulatory drugs are used. While the most common result in those cases is twins, a few women have even had septuplets as a result of fertility drugs.

Artificial insemination

By definition, artificial insemination involves the injection of sperm into the vagina or uterus by artificial means rather than through normal intercourse. Artificial insemination may use the husband's sperm (AIH) or donor sperm (AID). Often these procedures are lumped together under the term "intrauterine insemination" (IUI) to avoid the negative connotation sometimes associated with the term "artificial." Because AIH and AID are more familiar and descriptive, we will keep the procedures separate in our discussion. While the techniques are relatively simple, they are not without ethical concerns. We will discuss these below.

In vitro fertilization

In vitro fertilization (IVF) is a combined procedure using fertility drugs and egg transfer techniques *in vitro* (from the Latin, meaning "in glass," referring to the glass petri dish that is used). A woman's body normally releases one egg per month. Using fertility drugs, a doctor can make a woman release many eggs. Once the eggs are retrieved, they can be fertilized in a petri dish and the resulting embryos can be transferred to a woman's uterus.

An alternative procedure is called gamete intrafallopian transfer (GIFT). The procedure is performed just like IVF, except that the sperm and the unfertilized egg are transferred to a woman's fallopian tube where fertilization can take place. According to the latest nationwide data, GIFT is successful about 24.1 percent of the time, while IVF is successful in about 25.2 percent of cases.[4]

Another infertility treatment is zygote intrafallopian transfer or ZIFT. With ZIFT, the zygote, which is a very young embryo, is transferred to a woman's fallopian tube in hopes that the developing baby will make his or her way down the tube and implant in the uterus. ZIFT is successful in 26.9 percent of cases.

Embryo freezing
Once a woman's eggs have been retrieved and fertilized, the resulting embryos may be frozen for later use. Typically in IVF, about a dozen eggs

will be retrieved and fertilized. Only about 3 or 4 embryos will be transferred to the woman's uterus. The others will be frozen. In some cases, couples will either be unsuccessful and stop trying to get pregnant, or achieve the number of children they want. If they created more embryos than they used, those embryos may remain in storage indefinitely. It is estimated that there are somewhere between 100,000 and 150,000 so-called spare embryos in fertility clinics around the country. Some experts estimate that as many as 25 percent of frozen embryos do not survive the thawing process between the first and second rounds of embryo transfer.

Egg donation
This is the mirror image of AID. Instead of using donor sperm to achieve pregnancy, eggs are donated by a third party. Because some women cannot produce sufficient numbers of eggs or a sufficient quality of eggs, third party egg donors are sometimes enlisted. They may be paid as much as $80,000 to $100,000 for their eggs.

Surrogacy
Simply stated, surrogacy involves one woman becoming pregnant for another woman. The sur-

rogate mother may be inseminated by a man's sperm and be the egg donor herself. Or, an embryo resulting from IVF may be transferred to the surrogate's uterus. The surrogate may be a family member, a friend, or in some cases, a person who is paid to carry a couple's child to term.

Ethics of Reproductive Technologies

The growing number of reproductive technologies raises an equal number of ethical concerns. Only those technologies that pass ethical muster should be used. Some of the concerns to be considered include the sanctity of human life and the biblical ideal of the family.

Sanctity of human life
One of the biblical "realities" discussed in chapter 3 is the sanctity of every human life. At the moment human egg and sperm unite, a unique genetic individual is created. Individuals receive half their genetic identity from their biological mother and half from their biological father. Every human individual is created in God's image

> **S**ome of the concerns to be considered include the sanctity of human life and the biblical ideal of the family.

(Genesis 1:27) and is vested by God with inestimable value. As we have argued earlier, elective abortion is contrary to this biblical reality.

Some high-tech reproductive technologies do not by themselves violate the sanctity of human life. For example, IVF, AIH, GIFT, and ZIFT do not require that embryos be destroyed. They can, however, put embryos at risk, especially if combined with embryo freezing. Also, any time more than two or three embryos are implanted in a woman's uterus, there is a substantially higher likelihood one or more of those embryos will be put at risk of dying.

A further problem with creating extra embryos has to do with the impossibility of couples knowing what might happen between the time the embryos are created and the time they are implanted. Some will recall the famous legal battle *Davis v. Davis*. The Davises tried to use IVF and embryo freezing to achieve pregnancy. Before Mrs. Davis could get pregnant, the couple divorced. Mr. and Mrs. Davis disagreed vehemently about what should happen to the frozen embryos. After several very lengthy court battles going all the way to the Tennessee Supreme Court, the embryos were destroyed.[5]

This case also highlights how important it is for couples to consider all the possible scenarios they might experience in the course of assisted reproduction. Couples should be encouraged to discuss their religious and moral commitments with their doctor *before* they begin therapy. Once embryos are created they cannot be uncreated.

If the husband's sperm is required for assisted reproduction, the wife can certainly assist in the retrieval process. In some cases, men are given a sterile plastic vial and instructed to donate sperm via masturbation. Often pornography is made available in the clinic to stimulate arousal. Not only does this violate Jesus' command not to lust (Matthew 5:28), but it unnecessarily separates a husband and wife from the intimacy of procreation.

Ideal of the family in the Bible

Just as procreation is part of the biblical ideal for the family, so too is monogamous marriage. The apostle Paul was being completely consistent with this ideal when he cited Genesis in his instructions on the family in the book of Ephesians: "For this reason a man will leave his father and mother and be united to his wife, and the two will become one flesh" (Ephesians 5:31). God's ideal for the family is one man and one woman, in a one-flesh kind of union, for life. We all know from experience, whether through our own families or those around us, how traumatic it is when this ideal is violated by adultery, divorce, or even death. This ideal is to be preserved and practiced for the well-being of the family, even when considering reproductive technologies.

Where the biblical ideal for the family is violated, heartbreak typically follows. As we explained in chapter 3, acting contrary to God's created plan is asking for trouble. Abram and Sarai stand out as important examples. In fulfillment of his promise to Abram, God intended to give Abram and Sarai children—but on God's own timetable.

In their unbelief and impatience, Abram and Sarai decided to take matters into their own hands. "So [Sarai] said to Abram, 'The Lord has kept me from having children. Go, sleep with my maidservant; perhaps I can build a family through her' " (Genesis 16:2). Thus, Sarai offered her servant, Hagar, as an egg-donating surrogate—a violation of God's ideal for the family. Ishmael was born when Abram was eighty-six years old. As one might imagine, Sarai and Hagar's relationship deteriorated. "Then Sarai mistreated Hagar; so she fled from her" (Genesis 16:6). The result of violating God's ideal was heartache and disruption of the family. Later, in God's own time—when Abram was ninety-nine and Sarai was ninety—God caused Sarai to conceive and she bore a son and named him Isaac. While God graciously blessed Ishmael (Genesis 17:20), it was with Isaac that he established his covenant.

A number of the reproductive technologies violate God's ideal for the family and are, therefore, rife with difficulties. For instance, surrogate motherhood, one of the more controversial of the reproductive technologies, is contrary to the "nuclear" structure of the family. When a third party intrudes on the procreative relationship, the divinely instituted structure of the family is altered.

Commercial surrogacy—where a woman is paid to carry a couple's child to term—is the most objectionable form of surrogacy. The practice reduces children and childbearing to a form of barter. This practice makes reproduction little more than a commercial relationship and the surrogate little more than a womb for rent.

Even altruistic surrogacy, where no money changes hands, is problematic. Surrogacy works best when the surrogate mother is emotionally detached from the child she is carrying in her body. Yet, a child is better off when a mother is invested emotionally in her child and in her pregnancy. The conflict of interest works against the best interests of the child even in the case where a family member serves as a surrogate.

Furthermore, laws governing surrogacy arrangements are still evolving in many states. This fact makes surrogate motherhood far from ideal. Children need the very best environment for nurture, even *in utero*. Surrogacy fails to meet important criteria for compassionate child rearing. One possible exception to this is so-called "rescue surrogacy." In this arrangement, a woman agrees to carry and adopt an unwanted embryo who was frozen in a fertility clinic. At least one embryo adoption agency has been established to facilitate embryo adoptions (see www.snowflakes.org). Rescue surrogacy should not, however, be thought of as merely another form of reproductive technology. The practice would no longer be necessary once the unwanted embryos were all adopted.

Egg donation and artificial insemination using donor sperm also violate God's ideal for the family by creating a child who results from the union of the husband or wife and another person outside of the marriage. Unlike adoption—which "redeems" a child who would otherwise not have a family—these arrangements *create* a situation where the parents are not equally related to a child they bring into the world. They also expose children and adults to intensely traumatic challenges, both legal and otherwise.

A Theology of Infertility

When making procreative decisions, Christians have more than technological questions to ask. Reproductive technologies are not value-neutral. That is, just because these technologies are available does not mean that they ought to be used or that they pass ethical muster. Like other decisions, decisions concerning reproductive technology should be informed by a Christian worldview. What does the Bible say about infertility?

First, bearing children is good and parenthood is to be celebrated. From the beginning, God blessed procreation. In Genesis 1:28, God said:

"Be fruitful and increase in number; fill the earth and subdue it." Similarly, the psalmist says: "Children are a gift from the Lord; they are a reward from him. Children born to a young man are like sharp arrows in a warrior's hands. How happy is the man whose quiver is full of them! He will not be put to shame when he confronts his accusers at the city gates" (Psalm 127:3-5, NLT). Not insignificantly, "God sent his Son, born of a woman, born under law, to redeem those under law, that we might receive the full rights of sons" (Galatians 4:4). That is, God chose to use the procreative process to bring his Son into the world, albeit through the virgin giving birth. Not only that, but children occupied a special place in Jesus' ministry (see Matthew 18:1-6 and Mark 10:13-16). Furthermore, the believer's relationship to God is defined as a parent-child relationship: "The Spirit himself testifies with our spirit that we are God's children. Now if we are children, then we are heirs—heirs of God and co-heirs with Christ" (Romans 8:16-17).

Second, it is equally clear that the sovereign Lord is the one who opens and shuts the womb (1 Samuel 1:5-6). While children are clearly a blessing from God, the ability to bear them is subject to the mystery of his providence. In fact, the apostle James warns Christians not to be presumptuous about their lives. Rather than brazenly following our own desires, we are taught, "Instead . . . say, 'If it is the Lord's will, we will live and do this or that' " (James 4:15).

God's providence should not be a dark and foreboding reality for believers. As our Father, he always has his own glory and our best interests at heart—and there is never any conflict between the two. While we ought not cite the verse flippantly to people who are suffering, it is nonetheless true that "we know that in all things God works for the good of those who love him, who have been called according to his purpose" (Romans 8:28). God is able to work good through our tragedies and traumas. He is also eager to use technologies ethically employed—that is, operating in harmony with his purposes and character—to free us from difficult circumstances. One of the most assuring realities of the Christian faith is the *purposefulness* of God. He never makes mistakes, commits errors of judgment, or acts capriciously.

In some cases, it may not be God's will for a couple to have children. Infertile couples should not be made to feel like second-class humans because they cannot conceive. God may well have other good and gracious purposes for them.

Infertile couples should not be made to feel like second-class humans because they cannot conceive. God may well have other good and gracious purposes for them.

Sadly, many couples assume that infertility is always a sign of God's disfavor or a means of punishment. That is not necessarily the case. On the other hand, God's will may be to bring a couple through the experience of infertility before they conceive. Of one thing we can be certain, God has promised never to place more of a burden on us than we can bear (1 Corinthians 10:13).

Finally, trials, including infertility, are sometimes brought into believers' lives as an encouragement to pray. First Samuel 1 is a powerful reminder that prayer is often God's appointed means of fulfilling his purposes for us. Hannah was an infertile woman who desperately wanted a child. She was extremely depressed over her inability to conceive. She prayed so intensely that the priest thought she might be drunk. Hannah responded to his allegation by saying, "I am a woman who is deeply troubled. I have not been drinking wine or beer; I was pouring out my soul to the Lord" (1 Samuel 1:15). In time, Hannah conceived and she had a son she named Samuel ("heard of God" in Hebrew). God answered Hannah's prayers just as he answers all his children's prayers, by accomplishing his loving purposes in their lives.

Conclusion

Infertility can be very traumatic for couples. The array of reproductive technologies offered can be confusing. Decisions about which technologies to use take a great deal of mental, emotional, and spiritual effort. There are several important ways family and friends can help couples deal with infertility.

Be informed. Learn the facts about infertility. Infertility is not necessarily a life-long condition. Some couples may experience years of infertility before having children. Do not give unsolicited advice or repeat old fables. Stories about a family member or friend who was infertile but recently had a baby may not bring comfort to couples in the throes of dealing with their own infertility. There are a number of groups that specialize in helping infertile couples. Hannah's Prayer is a

Christian support network for infertile couples. Stepping Stones Ministry publishes a newsletter for infertile couples.[6]

Be sensitive. Special occasions, like Mother's Day, may be very difficult for infertile couples. Understand why they might not feel comfortable participating on those occasions. When you learn that a couple is experiencing infertility, do not ask "Whose fault is it?" Sometimes couples feel guilty about infertility in the first place. Additional feelings of guilt—either real or imagined—do not help.

Be supportive. Support infertile couples by praying for them, pointing them to good resources, and just bearing their sense of burden with them as they seek help for their infertility.

8 Send in the Clones?

There was a global gasp in 1997 when Ian Wilmut and his colleagues in Edinburgh, Scotland, first announced the cloning of an adult mammal—a Fin Dorset sheep named Dolly. Even though the cloning of Dolly was not entirely successful, that which could only be imagined as science fiction had become science fact. If one mammalian species could be cloned, surely the cloning of a human being could not be far off. As we now know, the cloning of a human being is a present reality. Not only are some egotistic scientists continuing their efforts to clone human beings, but Australian researchers have disclosed that they have already cloned human embryos. The clone age is here.

Explaining Our Unease with Cloning

The North American public is decidedly against cloning human beings. In nearly every poll, the overwhelming majority of those surveyed find the idea of cloning a human being repugnant. In a poll released by ABC's *Nightline* program the day after the Dolly announcement, 87 percent of those polled said the cloning of a human being should be banned. Eighty-two percent said cloning human beings would be morally wrong, and 93 percent said they personally would not choose to be cloned.[1] Surprisingly, opposition to human cloning has remained incredibly consistent despite the years that have passed since 1997 and the way media attention tends to desensitize people to news.

In an often-cited article in *The New Republic,* Leon Kass of the University of Chicago argued that cloning is not "to be fretted about for a while, but finally to be given our seal of approval . . . the future of our humanity hangs in the balance." Human cloning, he maintained, ought to be prohibited immediately.[2]

At the same time, some scientists have asked us to lower our defenses and give human cloning a shot. In an editorial in the same issue of *Nature* magazine that premiered Dolly, the cloned sheep, we were told that "Ethical constraints aside, there are even some rare genetic and medical disorders for which [cloning] would be a desirable way for a couple to produce offspring." President Clinton's temporary moratorium on human cloning was castigated in the same article: "At a time when the science policy world is replete with technology foresight exercises, for a U.S. president and other politicians only now to be requesting guidance about what appears in today's *Nature* is shaming."[3] The International Academy of Humanism, a group which includes such luminaries as Francis Crick, Richard Dawkins, Anthony Flew, W. V. Quine, Kurt Vonnegut, and E. O. Wilson, "call[ed] for continued, responsible development of cloning technologies, and for a broad-based commitment to ensure that traditionalist and obscurantist views do not irrelevantly obstruct beneficial scientific developments," which include human cloning.[4]

We might have anticipated such reactions. Boston University professor of health law, George Annas, pointed out a long time ago that "ethics is generally taken seriously by physicians and scientists only when it either fosters their agenda or does not interfere with it. If it cautions a slower pace or a more deliberate consideration of science's darker side, it is dismissed as 'fearful of the future,' anti-intellectual, or simply uninformed."[5]

Nevertheless, it is important to understand *why* human cloning is wrong.

Why Human Cloning Is Wrong

How was Dolly cloned? First, Ian Wilmut and his colleagues took a cell from an adult sheep's udder. They extracted the nucleus from the cell. The nucleus contains most of the DNA—the library of genetic information—in the cell. They then took a nucleus from the sheep they wanted to copy and inserted it in the host cell they had extracted. Because of the manipulation of the nucleus, the procedure is sometimes referred to as "somatic cell nuclear transfer." The Greek word "soma" means "body." Somatic cells are the body's cells other than sperm cells and egg cells. After transferring the nucleus to the host cell, researchers administered a very small electrical pulse and the cell began to divide just like any normal embryo. The cloned embryo was placed in a surrogate mother and some months later, *voilá,* Dolly was born! Only Dolly was not quite so normal. She grew to be much larger than other adult sheep, she showed signs of early aging, and developed premature arthritis. We have since learned that these are almost universal complications of cloned mammals.

Once they understand what cloning involves, the first question people usually ask about human cloning is: "Would a cloned human be a human person?" There is no good reason to assume that a human clone would be any less human than a person conceived through normal reproduction. A cloned human being would have the full complement of genetic information in her DNA. Clones would be a nearly exact copy of their original, so we could expect them to be persons just as the original is a person. If we take our experience with Dolly the sheep as an example, a cloned human being would possess all the qualities and faculties of any other human being.

From a Christian perspective, cloned human beings would be as much persons as any other human beings. They would be embodied souls and imagers of God (Genesis 1:27; 9:6). Humans are, according to Christian theology, the only beings made in the image of God (*imago Dei*). As imagers of God, human clones would possess the same dignity and divinely-bestowed moral value as any other members of our species. But that fact alone does not mean it would be right to clone a human being.

The dignity of individual human lives both prescribes and prohibits certain ways of treating human beings. For instance, human beings should not be used as means to our own ends. They should not be the subjects of experiments without their knowledge and permission. We

Human beings should not be used as means to our own ends.

may not demean human beings by imposing upon them harmful conditions to which

they have not consented. The experiments on Jews in Nazi Germany during World War II, the Tuskegee, Alabama, experiments on African Americans with syphilis, and Tennessee radiation experiments on unsuspecting workers have all been very painful lessons about how human beings should not be treated in research.

Based on these principles, most of the reasons that have been suggested as reasons to clone human beings are immoral. Thus, human clones would not be suitable "organ farms" for those needing transplantable organs. Human clones would not be acceptable "substitutes" for children who died leaving their parents grief-stricken. Likewise, humans should not be cloned as a form of self-worship by those who want more than one of themselves around for posterity.

Furthermore, doing research on human embryos for cloning is wrong in and of itself. Note that it took some 277 attempts to clone one little lamb. That means that 276 lamb embryos were sacrificed on the altar of biotechnology. While this might be an acceptable practice when cloning sheep (providing the sheep were not abused in the lab), such experimentation would be unconscionable when applied to human embryos.

Time magazine's February 19, 2002, pictorial, "How to Clone a Human," was absolutely chilling. The authors estimated that it might take 400 human ova (eggs) to start a full scale cloning operation. "According to experts," the caption says, "producing a single viable clone will require scores of volunteers to donate eggs and carry embryos—most of which will have major abnormalities and never come to term. The clones that do survive could suffer more subtle problems that might show up well after birth." Near the end of the chart there is an image of a "baby clone." Next to that image are images of two human babies surrounded by dotted lines (similar to the lines used to mark homicide victims on the floor of a crime scene) with the caption: "some babies do not survive." Even if the end were justifiable, the means would not justify the end.

Research on animal clones has demonstrated

that cloning humans would result in untold loss of life and grotesque consequences in the lives of those who survived. University of Hawaii researcher Ryuzo Yanagimachi has observed that "Cloned embryos have serious developmental and genetic problems."[6] Dr. Brigid Hogan, professor of cell biology at Vanderbilt University calls human cloning "morally indefensible," and Dr. Rudolph Jaenisch of Massachusetts Institute of Technology calls human cloning "reckless and irresponsible."[7] Jaenisch points out that if cloned embryos are created "most of those will die in utero. Those are the lucky ones. Many of those that survive will have . . . abnormalities."[8]

In the largest study to date, researchers at the Whitehead Institute found that cloned mice suffered from serious genetic defects resulting in premature death, pneumonia, liver failure, and obesity. So, merely from a safety standpoint, human cloning would be morally unconscionable and scientifically repugnant.

In the largest study to date, researchers found that cloned mice suffered from serious genetic defects.

Some have suggested that human beings should be cloned, but only allowed to develop to the embryonic stage before using them for research. Through this means, the embryos could be sources of genes, cells, or tissues for experimental purposes. As we saw in chapter 4, there is no relevant moral distinction between an embryo and a baby who has already been born. Because both are imagers of God, both possess the same dignity and deserve the same protection. *Embryo, baby,* and *adult* are merely three terms we use to distinguish between stages of biological development. These terms should not be used to obscure the moral implications of how we treat human lives at different stages of development. With respect to our species membership, these terms represent a distinction without a moral difference. All are human beings who deserve equal respect. Accordingly, creating embryonic clones in order to destroy them for research is even worse than creating them to be born, in that the harm done to them is intended rather than unintended.

A number of religious bodies have taken clear stances against human cloning. The Roman Catholic Church, the Southern Baptist Convention, and other denominations have called for a comprehensive ban on human cloning. Interestingly, even denominations that would not be considered traditionally "pro-life" have spoken out against cloning. For instance, the United Methodist Church's General Board of Church and Society concurs with this view. Their Genetic Science Task Force issued a statement on May 9, 1997, calling for a complete ban on human cloning, including any procedure that creates what they call "waste embryos." The Task Force's conclusion was very interesting: "As Christians, we affirm that all human beings, regardless of the method of reproduction are children of God and bear the Image of God. If humans were ever cloned, they along with all other human beings, would have inherent value, dignity, and moral status and should have the same civil rights."[9]

Cloning and the Family

Another major focus in the cloning debate is on the way human cloning would impact the family. Family is, obviously, a very important institution in Christian theology. Many have observed that human cloning would upset traditional family patterns.

Randolfe Wicker, one of the founders of the Mattachine Society, an early homosexual rights advocacy group, sees cloning as a desirable means of asexual reproduction. Jack Nichols, author of *The Gay Agenda: Talking Back to the Fundamentalists,* says, "Let's not rush to judgment and forget the way in which the technology might help gay people create their own families, free from the coercion of the state."[10] Men, of course, are the earlier potential losers here, since they would no longer be necessary for reproduction if it is done through cloning. If an artificial uterus is perfected, eventually women might not be necessary either.

Quite apart from the debate over homosexuality, cloning raises important questions: Why have children? Why reproduce? From a biblical perspective, childbearing within a monogamous heterosexual marriage is normative. From the beginning God said, "in the image of God he created them; male and female he created them" (Genesis 1:27) and "Therefore shall a man leave his father and mother, and shall cleave unto his wife, and they shall be one flesh" (Genesis 2:24, KJV). From this one-flesh relationship children proceed. They are "a heritage from the Lord," as the psalmist says. They are a gift from God. Procreation should not be viewed as a form of self-definition. Rather, bearing children is a covenant responsibility granted sovereignly by the God who made us.

Bearing children is a covenant responsibility granted sovereignly by the God who made us.

In the Bible there is a presumption in favor of procreation. We are told to "Be fruitful and increase in number; fill the earth" (Genesis 1:28). As Anglican theologian Oliver O'Donovan points out, "Some understanding like this is needed if the sexual relation of a man and woman is to be more than simply a profound form of play."[11]

Nevertheless, children are to be viewed as a divine gift, not a narcissistic means of self-definition. The gift of children comes with an enormous bundle of moral and spiritual obligations. Children are to be reared "in the training and instruction of the Lord" (Ephesians 6:4). They are not means to achieve our own goals, aspirations, or desires. They are entrusted to us by a good and gracious God.

Some forms of reproductive technology have separated fertility and childbearing from the procreative act, and in many cases from the marital relationship. This separation has great moral consequences. As Christian ethicist Gilbert Meilaender has said, "In our world there are countless ways to 'have' a child, but the fact that the end 'product' is the same does not mean that we have done the same thing."[12]

There are many additional concerns raised by human cloning, such as, to what extent do children have a right to expect to have a mother and father? Wouldn't family relationships be confused through cloning? Would a clone be a sibling or a child of the original? How do we combat the inherent eugenic motivations behind human cloning? Would persons with disease genes be cloned? Would the nearsighted, farsighted, or deaf be cloned? Would the obese or frail be cloned? That is, how would cloning be used to discriminate against individuals who may or may not measure up socially in any given era? Leon Kass may not be far off when he says of the cloning debate: "We must rise to the occasion and make our judgments as if the future of humanity hangs in the balance. For so it does."[13]

Conclusion

The temptation to manipulate another human life is almost irresistible to some. Former University of Kentucky reproductive physiologist, Panos Zavos, and his Italian colleague, Severino Antinori are, along with the Raelians, in a race to clone a human being. They doubtless believe they are more like Lewis and Clark than Dr. Jekyl or Dr. Frankenstein. They are nevertheless scientifically and ethically irresponsible.

The near inevitability of cloning does not, however, make it more welcome. We are exquisitely ill-equipped morally to deal with the reality of a human clone in our midst. Clones would first have to suffer the notoriety of being born through human somatic cell nuclear transfer. Next, their future would be shaped by someone else's past. That is to say, those who reared a clone would probably want to duplicate the environment of the donor as much as possible. Otherwise the experiment would be less likely to produce an identical replica of the original, since environment is as important as inheritance. So much for that celebrated quality called human freedom. Furthermore, proprietary interests would be at stake. Who owns a clone—the cloned, the clone, or the cloner? In the commodified world of biotechnology, the one with the most investment money is likely to win. So, obviously, the cloner would own the clone. Prospective parents might be able to purchase a clone, but the market would determine the selling price. And will the price be set in pounds, dollars, Euros, or yen?

In our view human cloning ought to be forthrightly banned or effectively postponed in order to engage in a global debate about the morality of human cloning. Critics of such a proposal say that the debate would prove intractable. Perhaps that fact alone is a necessary and sufficient reason to prohibit cloning a human being in the next twelve months, twenty-four months, or forever.

"I was convinced that there was still plenty of time." With those haunting words, Aldous Huxley looked back to the 1931 publication of his prophetic book, *Brave New World*. Huxley's vision of an oppressive culture of authoritarian control and social engineering was among the more shocking literary events of the twentieth century. But a mere twenty-seven years after the publication of his novel, Huxley was already aware that he had underestimated the threat of modern technocratic society. A technological threat to our culture and our humanity looms over us today in the form of human cloning and we do not have much time to act.

9 Who's Splashing in the Gene Pool?

The February 2001 publication of the first draft of the human genetic blueprint marked a new threshold in the genetic revolution. At long last a nearly complete dictionary of human genes was made available to the whole world. Understanding the language of our 30,000 genes leads to greater diagnostic power and may soon lead to increasing numbers of therapies and treatments for inherited diseases.

A Big Science Project

Most of us are aware of the power of our inherited genes. Eye color, hair color, and many other physical characteristics are linked to our genes. Genetic factors also have been linked to a host of major health problems and birth defects. Conditions such as cystic fibrosis, Duchenne's muscular dystrophy, Down's syndrome, Huntington's chorea, Alzheimer's disease, diabetes, cancer, and perhaps some forms of mental illness may each be traced to our genes. To date, little can be

done to treat, let alone cure, these diseases. However, through a major science project, funded by
U.S. tax dollars, we may someday be able to offer
treatments to help thousands of persons who suffer from these illnesses.

In 1990, the National Institutes of Health (NIH)
and the Department of Energy (DOE) officially
began a jointly sponsored initiative known as the
Human Genome Project (HGP). The HGP is a massive, 15-year project that has as one of its goals to
identify the sequence of the 3 billion base pairs of
DNA that together carry the complete human genetic blueprint. This genetic blueprint is known
as a "genome." By February 2001, we had a rough
draft of that blueprint.

The information generated by the Human Genome Project will be the source book for biomedical science in the 21st century and will be
of immense benefit to the field of medicine. It
will help us understand and eventually treat
many of the more than 5,000 genetic diseases
that afflict humankind, as well as the many
multifactorial diseases in which genes play an
important role.

Authorized by Congress in 1989, the HGP's
goals included (1) mapping and sequencing the

human genome, (2) mapping and sequencing the DNA of model organisms such as the fruit fly, (3) collecting and distributing available data, (4) examining the ethical, legal, and social issues of the project, (5) training researchers, and (6) developing and transferring genetic technologies for the worldwide effort. The budget for the HGP is more than $250 million per year, adjusted annually for inflation—that's over $3 billion total. This is big science!

For the first time in a major government-funded science project, 3 percent of the first five years' budget was set aside to study the ethical, legal, and social implications (ELSI) of the technology. The ELSI component of the project is critical because of the tremendous social and ethical implications of studying and manipulating human genetic material. The ELSI Working Group, a committee of scientists, ethicists, insurance professionals, and others asserted that, "Any scientific endeavor of this magnitude must be developed in concert with a plan to ensure that the public has access to the benefits in improved health care, which should be the result of the research. It is also imperative to protect individuals and society from possible hazards which may be a consequence of our improved ability to detect and predict hereditary illness. The use of genetic information, for good or ill, has long been an issue in our society. But the quantity and complexity of genetic information that should become available requires that special precautions be taken."[1]

The group correctly understood that this initiative carried with it responsibilities of monumental proportions. It is imperative that all of us understand as much as possible about the implications of the HGP and seriously reflect on what the Bible informs us about the ethics of such a study.

The HGP's accomplishments are already very promising. Genes have been isolated for a number of devastating illnesses, including amyotrophic lateral sclerosis (Lou Gehrig's disease), cystic fibrosis, Duchenne's muscular dystrophy, Fragile X syndrome, Huntington's disease, neurofibromatosis, retinoblastoma, retinitis pigmentosa, and Wilm's tumor. Announcements of the discovery of genes for

> It is imperative that all of us understand as much as possible about the implications of the Human Genome Project and seriously reflect on what the Bible informs us about the ethics of such a study.

other diseases are being made almost daily. Once the disease genes are identified, efforts can be made to find treatments or even cures for these diseases. Several genetic illnesses are already treatable through gene therapy.

The hope of being able to offer treatments and cures for genetically linked illnesses is absolutely wonderful. The relief of human suffering and the prospect of restoring health to those persons who are debilitated and die from these diseases is sufficient to endorse the project. Indeed, we should applaud and encourage scientists in their war against genetic illnesses.

Challenges for the Future of Genetic Medicine

The future of genetic medicine is also filled with social, ethical, and legal challenges, especially for the disabled community. Some of the most important challenges are highlighted below.

The diagnosis/therapy gap

While the ability to diagnose genetic conditions grows almost exponentially, there is a profound time gap between diagnosis and treatment. Sadly, to date there are very few effective therapies for genetically linked conditions. It is likely that for some time there will be many more genetic diseases diagnosed than can be treated.

This phenomenon has resulted in the emergence of a new class of patient: the presymptomatic ill. These are persons who have been diagnosed with a disease gene for which there is no treatment. In many cases they may not show symptoms of the disease for a number of years, sometimes never. Yet they carry the knowledge that they have a genetic condition that may one day lead to their disability or death.

No one knows what the psychological and social implications of the diagnostic/therapy gap will be. What might it be like for a young girl to know at eight years of age that she has the gene for Huntington's, a disease whose symptoms do not appear until forty or fifty years of age? How will that knowledge affect her life's choices? More importantly, how will that knowledge affect the choices of her parents as they nurture her? Will they be overprotective and smothering? Will they discourage long-term life planning?

Knowledge is power. Genetic knowledge is power to shape lives for good or ill. The challenge of genetic knowledge is knowing what to do with the information. For instance, women diagnosed with one of the breast cancer genes, BRCA-1 or BRCA-2, sometimes undergo prophylactic mastectomy because of their fear of getting cancer. In some cases, there was either misdiagnosis or misunderstanding of the meaning of the tests. The result is that some women experience unnecessary physical and psychological trauma associated with mastectomy. On the other hand, many women have doubtless dodged breast cancer by having the procedure. How do we balance the benefits and harms of genetic knowledge? This is a question with which we are only beginning to grapple.

> **The challenge of genetic knowledge is knowing what to do with the information.**

In an unscientific PBS online poll, only 62 percent of respondents said they would want themselves or a loved one to be tested for a gene that increases the risk for a disease. Twenty-six percent said they would not want the test. A full 11 percent say they do not know what they want.[2]

Confidentiality
Information about one's possible disease conditions is highly personal information. Individuals

may or may not want to know that information. Clearly there are others who might wish to have your personal genetic information, namely, your employer and your insurance company. After all, they, too, stand to lose if you become ill.

In 1982, only 1.6 percent of companies reported that they were using genetic tests for employment purposes. By 1997, the American Management Association found that the number had grown to about 10 percent of companies. Increasing numbers of persons report genetic discrimination in the workplace. They may be denied employment or promotions based on their genetic information. At the same time, only about twenty-one states have enacted laws to prevent workplace genetic discrimination and only forty-two states have even minimal protections against insurance discrimination based on genetic conditions.[3]

In that same PBS online survey, 93 percent said they thought employers should *not* have access to their employee's genetic information.[4] Poll after poll shows that overwhelming numbers of Americans want genetic privacy protected. Yet, there is no national comprehensive genetic privacy/anti-discrimination legislation.[5] What will the fu-

ture hold for those with genetic conditions? Will they
be able to get jobs? Will
they be able to secure insur-
ance? We should all contact our elected officials
to let them know our concerns about our national
genetic future.

What will the future hold for those with genetic conditions?

Prenatal screening
Another example of the power of genetic knowledge is its link to prenatal (before birth) genetic
screening. Prenatal screening may be performed
either before implantation or *in utero*. In
preimplantation screening, embryos are tested
for certain genetic conditions and either implanted or destroyed depending on the results
and wishes of the prospective parents. In
postimplantation screening, unborn children are
tested in the womb to see if they are carrying deleterious genes and then a decision is made either
to carry them to term or abort them.

Because of the diagnostic/therapy gap, almost
all prenatal genetic screening is used in connection with abortion decisions. Since there are so
few genetic therapies, prospective parents either
choose to bring children into the world with the

knowledge that they will carry a disease gene when they are born or parents may decide to terminate the pregnancy. The ethics of abortion has already been discussed in chapter 4. Some parents who would not choose embryo selection or abortion may refuse prenatal genetic testing, since they intend to bring a child to term regardless of genetic condition. Others may find the information important as they prepare for a child who may have disabilities. But who decides what is a disease gene and what is merely a different genetic condition? Rutgers University sociologist Marque-Louisa Miringoff has observed:

"In the pursuit of good health, we have begun to tread a fine line in 'human selection.' We often choose to rule out certain diseases or, more accurately, certain human beings with those diseases. In some cases, as with Tay-Sachs disease, an as of now invariably fatal illness in early childhood, such a decision may be motivated by compassion. From many viewpoints, there is little quality of life in any sense traditionally understood, and great anguish and tragedy.

"Other diseases, however, challenge our logic more severely; our sense of balance between cost and benefit is not clear. Huntington's chorea is a case in point. Would a Woodie Guthrie be born today? Would his parents, as carriers of the disease, bear a child with the known risk? Could we now or soon screen him out prenatally? If the pace of genetic intervention continues, such an individual would not be born. Yet, I for one, am glad that he lived, although I mourn the anguish of his later life. One wonders, too, whether some perception of his coming illness contributed to the extraordinary creativity of his life.

"Clearly, it is a just and meaningful desire to prevent fatal and debilitating diseases. Yet in pursuing this goal, we pay unobserved costs. In eliminating individuals with unwanted diseases, we also create a mind-set that justifies the process of human selection. We thus move into the questionable arena of human worth,

> **In eliminating individuals with unwanted diseases, we also create a mind-set that justifies the process of human selection.**

and to some degree eugenic thought. We forgo the idea of therapeutic change (that is, dietary change or other forms of treatment) and opt instead for elimination. Individuals are seen as flawed. It is easier and more desirable to prevent their existence than to work for their survival."[6]

A new eugenics

Eugenics is a compound word from two Greek words meaning "good" and "genes." The eugenics movement began at the turn of the twentieth century in England and the United States. Under the leadership of social engineers such as Francis Galton and Charles Davenport, the eugenics movement became a powerful social force.

So-called "Fitter Families" contests were held across the United States in the 1920s and 1930s. Fitter families were families with fewer incidences of physical and mental disability. Their ethnic heritage also had to remain intact. Racial intermarriage disqualified families. Thus, the fitter families were exclusively Caucasian. Mary T. Watts, cofounder of the first contest at the 1920 Kansas Free Fair, said: "While the stock judges are testing the Holsteins, Jerseys, and whitefaces in the stock pavilion, we are judging the Joneses, Smiths, and Johns." Winners were given a medal inscribed with the slogan, "Yea, I Have a Goodly Heritage."

The eugenics movement tried to create "better humans through breeding." Yet breeding was not the only way to achieve the desired goals. In order to prevent "undesirables" from reproducing, mandatory sterilization laws were enacted.

The "feebleminded," "indolent," and "licentious" were sterilized without their consent and sometimes against their expressed wishes. So-called "eugenical sterilizations" increased from around 3,000 in 1907 to over 22,000 in 1935. By the 1930s most states had mandatory sterilization laws. In one well-known case, a young mentally retarded girl named Carrie Buck was given the "choice" either to be sterilized or to be returned to an asylum. Because both her mother and grandmother had been mentally retarded, the famous jurist Oliver Wendell Holmes declared of Carrie Buck, "three generations of imbeciles is enough" and mandated that she be sterilized.[7]

With the power of genetic technology, a new eugenics has emerged. A 1992 March of Dimes poll found that 11 percent of parents said they would abort a fetus whose genome was predisposed to obesity. Four out of five would abort a fetus if the child would grow up with a disability. Forty-three percent said they would use genetic engineering if available, simply to enhance their child's appearance.[8]

Increasingly, college-age women are being solicited for their donor eggs on the basis of their desirable genetic traits. In the summer of 2000, the *Minnesota Daily,* the student newspaper of the University of Minnesota, ran an advertisement for egg donors. Preferred donors were women five foot six inches tall or taller, Caucasian, with high ACT or SAT scores, with no genetic illnesses, and extra compensation was offered to those with mathematical, musical, or athletic abilities. The ad stated that acceptable donors would be offered as much as $80,000 for their eggs.[9] This is eugenics with a vengeance.

Our culture's emphasis on the genetically "fit" and our difficulty in embracing those who are "less fit" fuels this new eugenics mindset. We must resist the new eugenicists if we are to preserve a truly human future.

For a Truly Human Future

To be sure, the genetic revolution will mean great advances in the relief of human suffering and the treatment of human diseases. We may even see genetic cures. At the same time, we must make informed and ethical choices about our genetic future.

Most people in the disability community already know that "disease" and "illness" are not value-free labels. Disabilities (like abilities) are largely social constructs rather than clear-cut categories. Unfortunately, many able persons and many in the scientific community seem unaware that this is the case.

Discrimination against persons because of their race, gender, or disability is an ugly reality. Discrimination based on genetic identity is even uglier. If we would see a truly human future for ourselves and for our children we must value individuals for who they are, not for what they can do. As imagers of God, every person should receive respect and be treated with dignity, regardless of their genetic condition.

Our laudable goal of treating human disease and relieving human suffering must not be allowed to become a tool for eliminating the *persons* who are suffering. To do so would be to use the good gift of genetic knowledge for evil ends. Only vigilance on the part of all of us can prevent a bleak genetic future. The social, ethical, and legal implications of the new genetics is not an arena for only the scientist, philosopher, theologian, or lawyer. We all have a stake in our genetic future.

Our laudable goal of treating human disease and relieving human suffering must not be allowed to become a tool for eliminating the *persons* who are suffering.

Where is God in Human Genetics?

What does the Bible say about genetic engineering? While the writers of the Old and New Testaments did not envision a scientific project like the HGP, the omniscient God who inspired them certainly foreknew and gave humans the capacity for such knowledge. All truth belongs to God and is ultimately given to us for his glory and for our good. There are both good uses and evil uses of the knowledge God reveals or enables us to discover, and our responsibility as stewards of this knowledge is to seek to use it in ways that will glorify God and bring good to humanity.

> **The omniscient God who inspired the biblical authors certainly foreknew and gave humans the capacity for genetic knowledge.**

Are there precepts, principles, or examples in Scripture that should shape Christian ethics with respect to genetic issues? Since we do not find the words *gene, genetics, or genome* in a concordance of the Bible, what are some of the scriptural principles which ought to inform our thinking about the Human Genome Project?

First, we must begin where the Bible begins—at creation. Human beings, like all of the universe, are the result of the creative activity of a personal

God. "In the beginning God created the heavens and the earth," declares Genesis 1:1. The doctrine of creation is the foundation of the Christian theistic worldview. Christians may not agree about or fully understand all of the particulars, but we begin with the conviction that the universe, including human life, is not the result of random events, the luck of the draw, or blind chance but the intentional action of an all-powerful, loving God.

Second, the Genesis account reveals that Adam and Eve, and all their progeny, were created in the image and likeness of God (Genesis 1:27). The human genome is, therefore, not only biologically unique, but spiritually (or metaphysically) unique. Human life has been invested by God with sacredness and has intrinsic value. Just as some ways of treating human life are clearly unethical and immoral, some ways of treating the most basic biological building blocks of human life are unethical and immoral.

Third, the Scriptures declare that when Adam and Eve sinned in the Garden of Eden, something tragic happened to the whole created order (Genesis 3:17-21; Romans 5:12). Though theologians characterize the results of the Fall differently, it is obvious to anyone who is observant that this is not the best of all possible worlds. Sin has brought with it disease and death. Not only that, but the fact that we human beings are sinners means we often find ways to use good things for evil purposes.

Since disease is ultimately the result of the corruption of the world through sin, it is critical that we understand that genetics will not be a new messiah to redeem us from all bodily or mental ills. At the same time, however, we ought to use genetic technology for the purposes of curing human disease where possible. The genome project is not, in and of itself, open to the charge of "playing God" any more than other medical therapies. Whenever we take advantage of medical therapies or interventions (even ones so common as aspirin or vaccinations) we are using technology to intervene against human disease.

There is, though, a curious reductionism that sees every human ill—physical, mental, or spiritual—as curable through genetics. Reducing the human predicament to "bad genes" makes the new genetics another utopian vision.

Fourth, we must acknowledge that all of God's creation, especially we humans, are "fearfully and wonderfully made" (Psalm 139:14). Efforts to better understand the human body, the disease process, and the ways to fight those diseases should, all things being equal, be celebrated and encouraged. Discovering more about the profound complexity of the human body, mind, soul, and spirit points to the reality of the Creator and gives believers more cause to praise and worship him intelligently. That our great God has permitted us to discover ways to relieve physical human suffering, save lives, and cure diseases is certainly a manifestation of his grace and mercy.

Some argue that we should go beyond merely curing human illnesses through genetics. In their view, people should be allowed to enhance future children by genetically altering sperm, egg, or any other initial cells from which children may some day develop. The notion of using genetics to enhance human beings is riddled with difficulties, particularly if children are designed from the beginning. For instance, doesn't the use of genetics to enhance our offspring lead us further down the path of treating our children as means to our own ends rather than ends in themselves belonging to God? We saw in chapter 2 where this kind of dangerous thinking leads. Furthermore, how can we be certain that our effort to enhance our children won't lead to unforeseen harmful consequences for them or future generations? It is one thing if people are consenting to risks that affect only themselves. Such is not the case here.

The problem is worse if the enhancements in view are not ones that every human being would obviously want. In that case, the absence of consent renders enhancement unethical. But even an enhancement that would be welcomed by all would be problematic, since only those who have significant financial resources would be able to afford it. We would likely end up creating a class system of genetic "haves" and "have nots."

Every good and perfect gift comes from God (see James 1:17). That fact makes it imperative that we neither misuse nor squander the gifts he gives, including the gift of genetic technology. Genetic science must be harnessed for human good, not human detriment.

Finally, we must face squarely the limits of the new genetics and not think more highly of it than it deserves. Genetics will not ultimately save us from death and the grave. Death remains an inevitability.

10 Remaking Humans: The New Utopians versus a Truly Human Future

If the nineteenth century was the age of the machine and the twentieth century the information age, this century is, by most accounts, the age of biotechnology. In this biotech century we may witness the invention of cures for genetically linked diseases, including Alzheimer's, cancer, and a host of maladies that cause tremendous human suffering. We may see amazing developments in food production with genetically modified foods that actually carry therapeutic drugs inside them. Bioterrorism and high-tech weaponry may also be in our future. Some researchers are even suggesting that our future might include the remaking of the human species. The next stage of human evolution, they argue, will be the post-human stage.

The New Utopians

Utopianism—the idea that we can enjoy a perfect society of perfect people on a perfect earth—is not new at all. Novelists, playwrights, social engineers, and media moguls have played with the idea for millennia. The new utopians, however, are a breed apart, so to speak. They are what we might call "techno-utopians" or "technopians." That is, they believe that technology is the key to the perfect society of perfect people on a perfect earth.

The new technopians actually have a name for themselves: transhumanists. According to the World Transhumanist Association:

Transhumanism (as the term suggests) is a sort of humanism plus. Transhumanists think they can better themselves socially, physically, and mentally by making use of reason, science, and technology. In addition, respect for the rights of the individual and a belief in the power of human ingenuity are important elements of transhumanism. Transhumanists also repudiate belief in the existence of supernatural powers that guide us. These things together represent the core of our philosophy. The critical and rational approach which transhumanists support is at the service of the desire to improve humankind and humanity in all their facets.[1]

Again, the idea of improving society through technology is not new. In fact, most of the last century was spent doing just that. What is new, however, is how the transhumanists intend to use technology. They intend to craft their technopia by merging the human with the machine. Since, as they argue, computer speed and computational power will advance a million fold between now and the year 2050 A.D., artificial intelligence will surpass human intelligence. The only way humans can survive is by merging with machines, according to the transhumanists. Do the movies *AI* or *Bicentennial Man* come to mind?

Now, before you dismiss the transhumanists as just another group of space-age wackos, you need to

The only way humans can survive is by merging with machines, according to the transhumanists.

know who some of them are. One of the brains behind the movement is a philosopher at Yale University, Nick Bostrom. Bostrom's Web site (www.nickbostrom.com) sets out his worldview quite clearly. He wants to make better humans through technology.

Another transhumanist is a professor of cybernetics at the University of Reading in England.

Kevin Warwick claims the distinction (?) of being the first "cyborg." He wears implanted computer chips in his arm and wrist. The next stage of human evolution, argues Warwick, is the cybernetic age. As Warwick told *Newsweek* in January 2001, "The potential for humans, if we stick to our present physical form, is pretty limited. . . . The opportunity for me to become a cyborg is extremely exciting. I can't wait to get on with it." And so he has.

Rodney Brooks, professor of robotics at MIT believes that through robotics we are reshaping what it means to be human. His recent book *Flesh and Machines* is an exploration of his worldview. For many of the transhumanists, human beings are merely what AI guru Marvin Minsky has called, "computers made of meat."[2] So, melding biological computers (the human brain) with silicon brains (computers) seems like a good thing to do.

What do the transhumanists all have in common? First, to be most charitable, they find the problem of human suffering, limitation, and death to be unacceptable. The technopian vision is of a pain-free, unlimited, eternal humanity. While their motivation may be commendable, the real question is whether the means to their goals are ethically justifiable.

Secondly, and less charitably, the transhumanists display what can only be called selfloathing. They are very perturbed by humanity and its finitude. The body and its limitations have become a prison for them and they want to transcend the boundaries of mortality. In their view, transhumanism offers the greatest freedom.

Thirdly, they are confident—even triumphalisitic—evolutionists. Theirs is not the Darwinian evolutionary view of incredibly slow, incremental progress of the fittest of the species. No, this is good old Western pull-ourselves-up-by-ourbootstraps, relatively instant, designer evolution. But, with all of our human frailties, are we going to make ourselves better through technology? Since we are so limited, error-prone, and bounded, we might just destroy ourselves! The problem of self-extinction worries a few of them, especially Nick Bostrom.

Robots and computers will, of course, never become human. Why not? Because being "one of us" transcends functional biology. Human beings are psychosomatic, *soulish* unities made in the image of God. The image of God is fully located neither in our brain nor our DNA. We are unique combinations of body, soul, and mind. We might quibble theologically about how best to describe the components of our humanity, but most Christians agree that we are more than the sum of our biological and functional parts.

The technopians, however, do not share our view of what it means to be human. Even though computers and robots may never become human beings, some will doubtless attribute to them human characteristics and—it is not inconceivable to imagine—human rights, including a right not to be harmed. One day it may be illegal to unplug a computer and so end its "life" at the same time that it is an ethical duty to unplug a human being whose biology has ceased to function efficiently.

The apostle Paul could identify with some of the transhumanist's concerns. He, too, found the limitations of our fallen humanity bothersome. In 2 Corinthians 4 and 5 he groans about this earthly tabernacle or tent. Paul longs to be freed from the suffering, the

> **O**ne day it may be illegal to unplug a computer and so end its "life" at the same time that it is an ethical duty to unplug a human being whose biology has ceased to function efficiently.

pain, and the finitude. Yet, his hope is not in his own abilities to transcend his humanity, but in God's power to transform Paul's humanity through redemption. He is confident that this mortality shall put on immortality—that we have a dwelling place not made with human hands, but eternal, and heavenly. Paul writes:

> But we have this treasure in jars of clay to show that this all-surpassing power is from God and not from us. We are hard pressed on every side, but not crushed; perplexed, but not in despair; persecuted, but not abandoned; struck down, but not destroyed. We always carry around in our body the death of Jesus, so that the life of Jesus may also be revealed in our body. For we who are alive are always being given over to death for Jesus' sake, so that his life may be revealed in our mortal body. . . . Therefore we do not lose heart. Though outwardly we are wasting away, yet inwardly we are being renewed day by day. For our light and momentary troubles are achieving for us an eternal glory that far outweighs them all. So we fix our eyes not on what is seen, but on what is unseen. For what is seen is temporary, but what is unseen is eternal.

Now we know that if the earthly tent we live in
is destroyed, we have a building from God, an
eternal house in heaven, not built by human
hands. Meanwhile we groan, longing to be
clothed with our heavenly dwelling, because
when we are clothed, we will not be found na-
ked. For while we are in this tent, we groan and
are burdened, because we do not wish to be
unclothed but to be clothed with our heavenly
dwelling, so that what is mortal may be swal-
lowed up by life. Now it is God who has made
us for this very purpose and has given us the
Spirit as a deposit, guaranteeing what is to
come. (2 Corinthians 4:7-11; 16-18; 5:1-5)

Much of what the transhumanists long for is
already available to Christians: eternal life and
freedom from pain, suffering, and the burden of a
frail body. As usual, however, the transhumanists—like all of us in our failed attempts to save
ourselves—trust in their own power rather than
God's provision for a truly human future with
him.

Finally, since the role of the prophet is to declare the Word of the Lord to his covenant people,
the church must mount a massive educational

ministry to help Christians understand biotechnology from a Christian worldview perspective. That is to say, since all truth is God's truth, and since we live in a world that faces the brave new world of biotechnology, Christians have an obligation to understand how God's revelation applies to those technologies.

This will mean that seminaries will have to equip ministers to address the ethics of genetic engineering, gene therapy, transgenics, xenotransplantation, stem cell research, and a growing number of other issues. Currently most seminaries provide only limited opportunities to address these difficult areas. This is unfortunate because these are, and will increasingly become, the context of thorny pastoral problems. Pastors are even now being asked to provide counsel regarding reproductive technologies, but few are prepared to help because they find themselves uninformed not only about the technologies, but also about how to think about them.

> **S**ince all truth is God's truth, and since we live in a world that faces the brave new world of biotechnology, Christians have an obligation to understand how God's revelation applies to those technologies.

Further, the church in her prophetic role must use her regular educational ministry to develop a Christian mind on these issues. Every church member has a stake in the biotechnology revolution. Bioengineered plants and animals are already sold in grocery stores, often without labeling. Gene therapy will increasingly become the standard of care for many illnesses. Attempts will soon be made to create biochips for transferring information into and out of the human brain. Nanotechnology promises to create machines the size of molecules that will perform complex functions and microsurgery inside the human body.

The speed at which these biotechnologies are being developed means that often technologies are developed ahead of ways to counteract misuse, failure, or accidents. For instance, the push to produce implantable brain chips providing a live connection to the Internet is huge. Yet without foolproof protections against electronic viruses, the destruction of people's brains that results will be a far greater tragedy than burned-out desktop computers. Similarly unsettling is the prospect of self-replicating microscopic robots (nanobots) mistakenly or intentionally released into the environment with the ability to recognize and destroy specific genetically-distinct racial or other groups. The risks to our future and our children's future increases significantly with the exponential growth of such technologies. We urge, therefore, that none of these technologies should be developed without appropriate fail-safe plans. Otherwise, we will be controlled by our technology rather than the other way around.

In sum, not only is biotechnology remaking the world, it may remake human beings. Unless there is a context for Christians to discuss these technologies within the framework of a biblical ethic, there is no hope that they will be able to **Not only is biotechnology remaking the world, it may remake human beings.** make informed decisions about the use of these technologies.

Lastly, through her prophetic role, the church must help shape public policy related to biotechnology. Each of these technologies will require laws or policies to regulate or in some cases (such as cloning a human being) outlaw their use. At this point relatively few Christians—and even fewer churches—are informed about these issues. More alarming, they do not know how to impact the public policy process. This must change if the church is to be a faithful prophet to her culture and to her members.

Recommendations for Prophetic Ministry in the Biotech Century

☐ To more faithfully fulfill their prophetic role, churches must make it a priority to teach Christian ethics in general, and bioethics in particular, in the regular educational ministry of the church. Church educators must rethink the educational ministry of the church and give increased attention to bioethical and biotechnological issues.

☐ Since all of these biotechnologies impact human beings positively or negatively, pastors should preach and teach what the Bible tells us about human nature in the light of creation, the Fall, redemption, and glorification.

☐ Christian colleges and seminaries must carve out either curricular or extracurricular opportunities for students to learn about the developments in biotechnology and learn the skills to interpret technologies from a Christian worldview perspective.

☐ Christian institutions and policy groups should increase dedicated funding and personnel resources for biotechnology policy, including international policy work.

☐ Christian students should be encouraged to pursue vocations in medicine, biotechnology, and the sciences. We can impact biotechnology at the local level by bringing our convictions to bear in our own vocations.

☐ Christians should financially support research, education, and policy efforts aimed at securing a truly human future.

The decisions we make as individuals, as a nation, and as a global community will have lasting implications for the future. Biotechnological momentum is gathering. Today's decisions about biotechnology will set wheels in motion that will radically affect our grandchildren and their children's children for either good or ill. We must bring a genuinely Christian worldview to bear on the issues facing this Brave New World. If we do not, who will? If not now, then when?

Conclusion: Where Do We Go from Here?

In the days ahead, the ethics of medicine is going to become more important, not less. The further we move from a Judeo-Christian, Hippocratic vision for medicine, the less likely we are to keep the priorities of medicine in their proper order. As resources become more scarce and as society becomes increasingly preoccupied with whatever promises the biggest benefits, the more difficult it will become to treat patients as persons. As further reasons are offered for using human embryos in experimentation, the more difficult it will become for people to resist using unborn human beings as farms from which to harvest the vast natural resources they embody. As techniques for treating infertility continue to emerge, sorting among the various options will become more bewildering.

On the other hand, if medicine and biotechnology can be shepherded in directions that protect and promote human dignity, the future may be bright. God has called us to cultivate the earth as good stewards of God's good and gracious gifts.

Good stewardship demands faithfulness to God's revelation of himself in Scripture and attention to the priorities he has established. The first and greatest commandment—to love the Lord with all our hearts, souls, minds, and strength—requires that we devote our best efforts to develop medicine and biotechnology that will bring glory to our Maker.

If medicine and biotechnology can be shepherded in directions that protect and promote human dignity, the future may be bright.

Technology harnessed to biblical priorities has revolutionized human life throughout the centuries. In fact, the Christian worldview was instrumental in the growth and development of Western science and medicine. The second commandment—to love our neighbors as ourselves—calls on us to employ medicine and biotechnology for human healing for the good of the patient. Jesus' healing ministry provides a living example of the warrant for using our knowledge, skills, and technology for the relief of human suffering and the restoration of God's created order. Medicine and biotechnology, in service to God and human well-being, are powerful ways to worship God and minister to others.

The future has not yet been written. It is not only Christian physicians, nurses, other health care workers, clergy, ethicists, theologians, and scientists who have an important role to play in influencing the direction medicine and biotechnology take in the remainder of this century. Everyone—whether politician, voter, patient, or loved one helping with a health care decision—can and must make a difference!

Recommended Resources

Do you want to know more about bioethics from a Christian perspective? Whether you want to be connected with a network of Christians who are interested in medicine, biotechnology, and ethics, or you just want additional materials for your own study, resources are available to assist you. Contact The Center for Bioethics and Human Dignity, as explained on the page opposite the title page at the front of this book.

Here are some books to get you started (items marked with an asterisk [*] may be ordered at www.cbhd.org):

Hippocratic Health Care

* Cameron, Nigel M. de S. *The New Medicine: Life and Death After Hippocrates*. Rev. ed. Chicago: Bioethics Press, 2001.
* Stewart, Gary P., et al. *Basic Questions on Everyday Health Care*. Grand Rapids, Mich.: Kregel, 2003.
  Temkin, Owsei and C. Lilian, eds. *Ancient Medicine: Selected Papers of Ludwig Edelstein*. Baltimore, Md.: Johns Hopkins University Press, 1994.

Beginning of Life Issues

Alcorn, Randy. *ProLife Answers to ProChoice Arguments*. Sisters, Ore.: Multnomah, 2000.

Beckwith, Francis J. *Politically Correct Death: Answering Arguments for Abortion Rights*. Grand Rapids, Mich.: Baker, 1993.

Preece, Gordon, ed. *Rethinking Peter Singer*. Downers Grove, Ill.: InterVarsity Press, 2002.

Health Care Resources

* Kilner, John F. *Life on the Line: Ethics, Aging, Ending Patient's Lives, and Allocating Vital Resources*. Bannockburn, Ill.: The Center for Bioethics & Human Dignity, 2001.

* Kilner, John F., Robert D. Orr, and Judith Shelley, eds. *The Changing Face of Healthcare: A Christian Appraisal of Managed Care, Resource Allocation, and Patient-Caregiver Relationships*. Grand Rapids, Mich.: Eerdmans, 1998.

* Mitchell, C. Ben, Robert D. Orr, and Claretta Dupree, eds. *The Ethics of Aging and Life-Extending Technologies*. Grand Rapids, Mich.: Eerdmans, 2003, forthcoming.

End of Life Treatment

* Kilner, John F., Arlene B. Miller, and Edmund D.

Pellegrino, eds. *Dignity and Dying: A Christian Appraisal*. Grand Rapids, Mich.: Eerdmans, 1996.

Orr, Robert, David Biebel, and David Schiedermayer. *More Life and Death Decisions: Help Making Tough Choices about Care for the Elderly, Euthanasia, and Medical Treatment Options*. Grand Rapids, Mich.: Baker, 1997.

* Stewart, Gary P., et al. *Basic Questions on End of Life Decisions*. Grand Rapids, Mich.: Kregel, 1998.

Assisted Suicide and Euthanasia

Demy, Timothy J. and Gary P. Stewart, eds. *Suicide: A Christian Response*. Grand Rapids, Mich.: Kregel, 1998.

* Dyck, Arthur J. *Life's Worth: The Case Against Assisted Suicide*. Grand Rapids, Mich.: Eerdmans, 2002.

* Stewart, Gary P., et al. *Basic Questions on Suicide and Euthanasia*. Grand Rapids, Mich.: Kregel, 1998.

Reproductive Technologies

Evans, Debra. *Without Moral Limits: Women, Reproduction, and Medical Technology*. Rev. ed. Wheaton, Ill.: Crossway, 2000.

* Kilner, John F., Paige C. Cunningham, and W. David Hager, eds. *The Reproductive Revolution: A Christian Appraisal of Sexuality, Reproductive Tech-

nologies, and the Family. Grand Rapids, Mich.: Eerdmans, 2000.

* Stewart, Gary P., et al. *Basic Questions on Sexuality and Reproductive Technology*. Grand Rapids, Mich.: Kregel, 1998.

Genetic Engineering

* Kilner, John F., Rebecca D. Pentz, and Frank E. Young, eds. *Genetic Ethics: Do the Ends Justify the Genes?* Grand Rapids, Mich.: Eerdmans, 1997.

Song, Robert. *Human Genetics: Fabricating the Future*. Nashville: Darton, Longman & Todd, 2002.

* Stewart, Gary P., et al. *Basic Questions on Genetic Intervention, Stem Cell Research, and Cloning*. Grand Rapids, Mich.: Kregel, 2003.

Cloning, Biotechnology, and a Truly Human Future

* Cameron, Nigel M. de S., Scott E. Daniels, and Barbara J. White, eds. *BioEngagement: Making a Christian Difference Through Bioethics Today*. Grand Rapids, Mich.: Eerdmans, 2000.

* Kilner, John F., C. Christopher Hook, and Diann B. Uustal, eds. *Cutting-Edge Bioethics: A Christian Exploration of Technologies and Trends*. Grand Rapids, Mich.: Eerdmans, 2002.

* Kilner, John F., Nigel M. de S. Cameron, and David

L. Schiedermayer, eds. *Bioethics and the Future of Medicine: A Christian Appraisal.* Grand Rapids, Mich.: Eerdmans, 1995.

Journal Resource

∗ *Ethics and Medicine: An International Journal of Bioethics.* Published three times per year. (www.ethicsandmedicine.com) The journal is available directly or as part of membership in The Center for Bioethics & Human Dignity. The mission of *Ethics and Medicine* is to reassert the Hippocratic consensus in medicine as seen through the lens of the Judeo-Christian tradition, on the conviction that only a robust medical professionalism is able to withstand the challenges of emerging biotechnologies and their clinical applications.

Discussion Questions

Chapter 1

1. Briefly describe medical practices in ancient Egypt. How did Egyptian medical practices compare to those in Mesopotamia?
2. How did the Greeks influence scientific medicine?
3. If you had lived in ancient times, do you think you would have sought medical care as readily as you do today? Why or why not?
4. What is your first impression of the Hippocratic Oath? To what extent does it still apply to today's medical practice?
5. Explain "do no harm" in modern day terms. Has this changed since Hippocrates' time? How?
6. Does your family doctor follow the points of the Hippocratic Oath? Why is that important to you?
7. Have you or anyone in your family experienced questionable medical care? How did it affect the outcome of your treatment? What did you do about it?
8. How can ignoring the principles in the Hippocratic Oath jeopardize the well-being and care of patients?

9. What are some of the changes in the Oath that greatly affect medical ethics?

10. From a Christian viewpoint what do you think about the changes to the Oath mentioned in this chapter?

Chapter 2

1. How has the Hippocratic orientation of medicine changed in the past forty years?

2. "Bioethics from a Christian perspective not only can critically evaluate the ways that people justify their actions, but also can explain how people should live." Do you agree? Why or why not?

3. What are the four reasons that people arrive at different ethical conclusions? Which of the four most influences you and your ethical decisions?

4. Have you ever persuaded someone to change his or her opinion about an ethical issue? Have you been persuaded to change *your* opinion on an issue? In either instance, what influenced the change?

5. What are three approaches to reasoning? Which, if any, do you use most frequently?

6. What makes reasoning that appeals to consequences unworkable? Have you tried using that type of reasoning? What happened?

7. When are "right and wrong" not right and wrong?

8. Explain "bioethics of principles." What do some people consider the only absolute principle?
9. What are the shortcomings of autonomy ethics?
10. What are the limitations of following a "bioethics of virtues"?

Chapter 3

1. What are the three central characteristics of biblical bioethics?
2. What is meant by the phrase "God-centered bioethics"? What are the differences between it and a human-based bioethics?
3. What is sin? Does your understanding of it agree or disagree with the view in this chapter? Why do you agree or disagree?
4. Why do all people need God's help and direction for right thinking? What sort of direction does God provide us?
5. Why do we need to be realistic in our thinking and decision making? What are some of the results of being unrealistic?
6. What are some examples of reality that God alerts us to in the Bible—past, present, and future?
7. Which are the two great commandments according to Jesus? How are they the essence of what the Bible teaches? Which of these two commandments do you find most difficult to follow?
8. How did Paul make love-impelled decisions con-

cerning Titus and Timothy? How could they both be love-impelled and have the opposite conclusions?

9. How does the biblical approach compare with the approaches discussed in chapter 2? What is the weakness of each of the other (non-biblical) approaches?

10. How can recognizing the similarities and differences between a biblical bioethics and other popular approaches to bioethics be helpful?

Chapter 4

1. Describe a stem cell. How are the three types of stem cells used in research different?

2. "The great appeal of stem cell research is that there is ample evidence it will lead to cures or the treatments for many medical conditions." Has anyone you know benefited from receiving stem cells? Briefly discuss the circumstances and the results.

3. What are the ethical problems with using embryonic stem cells? What are the medical risks of using these cells? Why do people persist in pursuing this research?

4. How would you define an embryo? Does knowing that an embryo is a highly sophisticated entity change your thoughts about stem cell research? Why or why not?

5. Name six different points after fertilization at which some people think human beings first come into existence. What is wrong with the rationale given for each point?

6. What does the Bible have to say about embryos? How could you use these Scriptures to press the point that embryos are human beings? Have you ever been in such a discussion? What was the outcome?

7. If you or a family member had a disease that could be helped or cured by using stem cells, would you allow the treatment? Would you question where the stem cells came from? What would you do if you found they came from an embryo?

8. What are the ramifications of using fetal stem cells? In what instances is this an ethically acceptable option?

9. How can the term "bearing one another's burdens" be important in a discussion about stem cell research?

10. What were your thoughts and feelings about stem cell research before you read this chapter? Did the information in this chapter change your view? If so, how?

Chapter 5

1. Have you had a family member who was going through the process of dying and decisions about

his or her care needed to be made? Who made the decisions? How did you or other family members make these decisions? What were the results of your decisions?

2. How can life-sustaining technologies be a "double-edged sword"?

3. How do people who approach life with a focus on consequences, resolve end-of-life situations? What makes this approach dangerous and impractical?

4. How do those with an autonomy-based outlook view end-of-life decisions? What is dangerous about this view?

5. What is a biblical approach to a person's dying?

6. How do you define death? What does the Bible call death? What are the practical implications of seeing death as a defeated enemy?

7. Do you agree with this statement, "If continued life is not a possibility, then patients should receive only treatment that supports rather than burdens them in the dying process"? Why or why not?

8. What are the four important ethical safeguards that insure that what patients say reflects their true wishes?

9. Discuss the differences between a "living will" and a "durable power of attorney for health care." Why is it important for people to have these documents in place before they are needed? Do you or your family have either of these documents?

10. As a Christian, how can you promote the biblical justice that typically requires that all who want and need a scarce treatment should be given equal opportunity to receive it?

Chapter 6

1. What three parties are present in the room of any patient where end-of-life decisions need to be made? What stake does each have in the decision being made? In your opinion, which party is least likely to be considered? Why?

2. Have you known anyone who attempted suicide (successfully or unsuccessfully)? What emotions are brought forth by such an act? How would you counsel someone considering suicide?

3. Define assisted suicide. Why would someone seek another person's assistance to commit suicide?

4. How is physician-assisted suicide contradictory to what health care stands for?

5. What are the four major ways in which patients need support near the end of their lives? How can a patient be seduced by the thought of assisted suicide if even one of these supports is missing?

6. In what ways does assisted suicide violate biblical principles concerning life and God's love for all human beings?

7. Define the difference between assisted suicide and

euthanasia. What are the reasons given for euthanasia being used?

8. What has happened in countries where euthanasia is legalized? What is the very dangerous next step that can come from legalized euthanasia?

9. Which group of people is most at risk if euthanasia becomes more accepted and widespread?

10. As a Christian what can you do to counteract assisted suicide and euthanasia? Why is compassion an important factor?

Chapter 7

1. What do the authors mean with the term "low-tech" pregnancy? What practical guidelines are given to help achieve pregnancy in this way?

2. Briefly explain each of the following terms: fertility drugs, artificial insemination, in vitro fertilization, embryo freezing, egg donation, and surrogacy. With which of these are you most familiar? Which one(s) would you be most comfortable using or recommending to a friend?

3. What are the two types of artificial insemination? Do you find one preferable to the other? Why or why not?

4. What, if any, reservations would you have about using in vitro fertilization and embryo freezing? How about egg donation?

5. Put yourself in this scenario: You and your spouse are an infertile couple that has tried many methods to become pregnant but nothing worked. Would you try surrogacy? If not, why not? If so, whom would you choose to be the surrogate mother, and why would you choose that person?

6. What are some of the problems associated with creating embryos that are not used? How does this go against the sanctity of life?

7. What is the ideal of the family in the Bible?

8. Why is surrogate motherhood contrary to the "nuclear" structure of the family? How can it have negative effects on the child being carried? What is "rescue" surrogacy?

9. In what ways do egg donation and donor artificial insemination violate God's ideal for a family?

10. The authors list three ways family and friends can help couples deal with infertility. Do you know someone who could use your help? How would these suggestions be helpful to you?

Chapter 8

1. What was your reaction to the news in 1997 that a sheep had been cloned? How do you feel when you read about or hear discussions concerning human cloning?

2. Why are most surveyed people against human

cloning? Do you agree with their arguments? Why or why not?

3. What are some of the medical arguments against human cloning? What are the worst implications of making a viable human clone?

4. How could human cloning impact the family? How would the cloning of humans go against biblical ideals for family?

5. If a clone were made from you, would it be your child or your sibling?

6. How could human cloning be used to discriminate against some segments of society?

7. "The future of a cloned individual would be shaped by someone else's past." How do you interpret that statement? Do you agree with it?

8. Whom do you believe would own the cloned individual? Why?

9. How can human cloning pose a technological threat to our culture and our humanity?

10. If it were possible, would you want to be cloned? Give your reasons.

Chapter 9

1. List some of the physical attributes that are linked to our genes. What are some of the health problems that have also been linked to our genes?

2. What are the goals of the Human Genome Project?

Do you feel these goals are worth the tremendous amount of money being spent? Explain your response.

3. The genes that cause a number of devastating illnesses have been identified and some genetic illnesses are already treatable through gene therapy. But there is a profound time gap between diagnosis and treatment. What makes this "diagnosis/therapy gap" a cause of concern and frustration?

4. Define presymptomatic ill patients. If you found out that your young child has the gene for an illness that may affect her in middle age, how would you treat her? How would you counsel her as she matures and makes long-term plans?

5. Would you want to be tested for a gene that increases the risk for a disease? Why or why not? How would you make long-term plans if you knew that you *did* have the gene that put you at risk for a disease?

6. What are the dangers of prenatal screening? With what options may prospective parents be presented? Have you or anyone you know faced this dilemma? How was it resolved?

7. Briefly explain the term *eugenics*. How was it used in the 1920s and 1930s?

8. A new eugenics has emerged today—what is it? How is it different from eugenics of the '20s and '30s? How are its effects similar?

9. Genetics is not mentioned by name in the Scriptures but numerous Bible passages suggest scriptural principles, which ought to inform our thinking about the subject. Briefly discuss the four principles identified by the authors.

10. Read the final paragraph of this chapter. How can this be a statement of Christian faith?

Chapter 10

1. Give examples of the "age of biotechnology." How does it impact your everyday life?

2. Describe a transhumanist. Had you heard of the term before you read this chapter? Give your opinion of transhumanist goals and beliefs.

3. Making better humans through technology, cybernetic age, and robotics are the concepts of some transhumanists. Which, if any, sound interesting or appealing to you? Which seem "far-out" if not repulsive or alarming? Give reasons for your opinions.

4. What three things do all transhumanists have in common?

5. Why will robots and computers never become human? Why is this important to us as Christians?

6. Why do Christians have an obligation to understand how God's revelation applies to the brave new world of biotechnology?

7. How can Christian churches help their members in their understanding of biotechnology and how to make biblical decisions concerning these issues?

8. What is done in your denomination or local congregation to address biotechnology? If nothing is being done, what action can you take to make people aware of the opportunities and perils of a biotech world?

9. Do you agree with the recommendations listed at the end of the chapter? If you were writing these recommendations, would you add more or subtract some? Explain your answer.

10. How can decisions made today affect our children "unto the third and fourth generation?"

Notes

Introduction

1. Bill Joy, "Why the Future Doesn't Need Us," *Wired* vol. 8, no. 4 (April 2000).

Chapter 1: It Started with Hippocrates

1. Plato, *Phaedrus* 270 C–D.
2. Cited in Logan Clendening, ed., *Source Book of Medical History* (New York: Dover Publications, 1960), 15.
3. Nigel M. de S. Cameron, *The New Medicine: Life and Death After Hippocrates,* rev. ed. (Chicago: Bioethics Press, 2001), 32.
4. Hippocrates, *Epidemics* I, 11.
5. Robert Orr, Norman Pang, Edmund Pellegrino, and Mark Siegler, "The Use of the Hippocratic Oath: A Review of 20th Century Practice and a Content Analysis of Oaths Administered in Medical Schools in the U.S. and Canada in 1993," *The Journal of Clinical Ethics* 8 (4): 377–88.
6. Ibid.

Chapter 4: Embryonic Ethics

1. These studies are reported in *New Scientist* (26 January 2002) and *The New England Journal of Medicine* (7 March 2002).

2. For statistics and other information on the human genetic code, see the "Human Genome Project Information" Web site maintained by the U.S. Department of Energy at <http://www.ornl.gov/hgmis>.

Chapter 7: Thirty-eight Ways to Make a Baby

1. Bruce Albrecht, M.D., and Isaac Schiff, M.D., *The Office Practice of Medicine*, 3rd edition, ed. William T. Branch (Philadelphia: W. B. Saunders, 1994).
2. American Society of Reproductive Medicine.
3. Albrecht and Schiff, *Office Practice of Medicine,* 516.
4. Current statistics on all assisted reproductive technologies can be found on the Centers for Disease Control's Web site at <http://www.cdc.gov/nccdphp/drh/ART00/index.htm>.
5. Davis v. Davis (1990) Tennessee Appeals Court.
6. For more information on Hannah's Prayer, see <http://www.hannah.org>. You can find Stepping Stones Ministry at <http://www.bethany.org>.

Chapter 8: Send in the Clones?

1. ABC *Nightline* poll, *Nightline* Web site, the day after the Dolly announcement.
2. Leon R. Kass, "The Wisdom of Repugnance: Why We Should Ban the Cloning of Humans," *The New Republic* (2 June 1997): 18.

3. Editorial, "Caught Napping By Clones," *Nature* 385 (27 February 1997).

4. Press release, International Academy of Humanism, "Statement in Defense of Cloning" (16 May 1997).

5. George J. Annas, "Who's Afraid of the Human Genome?" *Hastings Center Report* (1989): 21.

6. Reuters News Service, "Report Says Scientists See Cloning Problems," 24 March 2001.

7. Ibid.

8. Jeremy Manier, "Potential Perils Born in Cloning," *Chicago Tribune*, 4 March 2001.

9. Statement from the United Methodist Genetic Science Task Force, General Board of Church and Society of the United Methodist Church, Washington, D.C. (9 May 1997).

10. Chris Bull, "Send in the Clones," *The Advocate* (15 April 1997): 37.

11. Oliver O'Donovan, *Begotten or Made?* (Oxford, 1984): 74.

12. Gilbert Meilaender, *Bioethics: A Primer for Christians* (Grand Rapids, Mich.: Eerdmans, 1996): 15.

13. Leon Kass, 18.

Chapter 9: Who's Splashing in the Gene Pool?

1. *Understanding Our Genetic Inheritance, The U. S. Human Genome Project: The First Five Years FY*

1991–1995 (National Institutes of Health Publication No. 90-1590, April 1990). Information about the Human Genome Project may be found at <www.genome.gov>.

2. <www.pbs.org/wgbh/nova/genome/survey.html>
3. For these data and other helpful information about genetic privacy see <http://www.gene-watch.org/programs/privacy.html>
4. <www.pbs.org/wgbh/nova/genome/survey.html>
5. For information on pending genetic legislation see <http://thomas.loc.gov> and enter keywords: "genetic privacy" or "genetic discrimination."
6. Marque-Louisa Miringoff, *The Social Costs of Genetic Welfare* (Piscataway, N.J.: Rutgers University Press, 1991), 159–60.
7. <www.eugenicsarchive.org/eugenics>
8. March of Dimes Birth Defects Foundation, *Genetic Testing and Gene Therapy: National Survey Findings* (White Plains, N.Y.: March of Dimes, September 1992).
9. *Minnesota Daily* (July 2000).

Chapter 10: Remaking Humans

1. <www.transhumanism.com>
2. Marvin Minsky cited in Gary Mar, "Can Computers Think?" *New Oxford Review* (December 1990): 27.

Topical Index

About the Authors

John F. Kilner is the president and CEO of The Center for Bioethics and Human Dignity in Bannockburn, Illinois. Author of numerous articles in medical, public health, legal, religious, and ethics journals, he has written or edited twelve recent books, including *Life on the Line: Ethics, Aging, Ending Patients' Lives, and Allocating Vital Resources,* and *Cutting Edge Bioethics: A Christian Explanation of Technologies and Trends.*

C. Ben Mitchell is Associate Professor of Bio- ethics and Contemporary Culture at Trinity International University in Deerfield, Illinois. He also serves as bioethics consultant for the Ethics and Religious Liberty Commission, the moral concerns, public policy, and religious liberty agency of the Southern Baptist Convention. He is a Fellow of The Council on Biotechnology Policy and a Senior Fellow of The Center for Bioethics and Human Dignity, where he serves as editor of the Center's international journal, *Ethics and Medicine: A Christian Perspective on Bioethics.*

Vital Questions
CLEAR THINKING FOR FAITHFUL LIVING

□ □

The Vital Questions series investigates key issues that make a practical difference in how Christians think and act. Each book's goal is to provide substantial, accessible discussion of issues about which Christians need to know more.

Look for the Vital Questions series wherever fine Christian books are sold.

Is God Intolerant?
by Dan Taylor

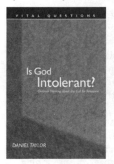

In contemporary culture, Christians have been called intolerant for standing up for what is right, for witnessing to other people about Jesus, and for stating that Jesus is the only way to God. In this volume, Dan Taylor, professor at Bethel College, explores the concept of tolerance. With depth and precision, he explains what true tolerance is and whether God wants Christians to be tolerant.

How *Shall* We Worship?
by Marva J. Dawn

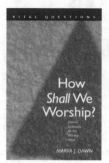

If your church is like most churches, you have debated the value of various types of worship styles in your service—traditional versus contemporary, hymns versus praise songs. It's too easy for people to take sides in the worship wars. Marva Dawn will help you understand why there are so many disagreements in the church about worship. You'll never view worship the same after reading this book.

Does God Need Our Help?
by John F. Kilner and C. Ben Mitchell

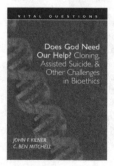

Cloning. Assisted Suicide. Stem Cell Research. The advance of biotechnology today is breathtaking. But do we know where all of this is leading us? John F. Kilner and C. Ben Mitchell will lead you on a fascinating journey, explaining the cutting-edge advances in biotechnology. This book will help you formulate an informed and thoroughly Christian perspective on everything from assisted suicide to infertility treatments, from cloning to stem-cell research.